Rodolfo Saracci

EPIDEMIOLOGY

A Very Short Introduction

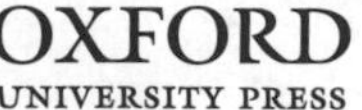
OXFORD UNIVERSITY PRESS

OXFORD
UNIVERSITY PRESS

Great Clarendon Street, Oxford OX2 6DP

Oxford University Press is a department of the University of Oxford.
It furthers the University's objective of excellence in research, scholarship,
and education by publishing worldwide in

Oxford New York

Auckland Cape Town Dar es Salaam Hong Kong Karachi
Kuala Lumpur Madrid Melbourne Mexico City Nairobi
New Delhi Shanghai Taipei Toronto

With offices in

Argentina Austria Brazil Chile Czech Republic France Greece
Guatemala Hungary Italy Japan Poland Portugal Singapore
South Korea Switzerland Thailand Turkey Ukraine Vietnam

Oxford is a registered trade mark of Oxford University Press
in the UK and in certain other countries

Published in the United States
by Oxford University Press Inc., New York

First published 2010

British Library Cataloguing in Publication Data
Data available

Library of Congress Cataloging in Publication Data
Data available

Typeset by SPI Publisher Services, Pondicherry, India
Printed in Great Britain by
Ashford Colour Press Ltd, Gosport, Hampshire

ISBN 978-0-19-954333-5

3 5 7 9 10 8 6 4

To Estelle.
Every newborn child is a hope
for a better world.

Contents

Preface

Health is everybody's natural concern, and an everyday theme in the media. Outbreaks of disease such as the most recent influenza, occurring in many countries at the same time, make front-page news. Beyond epidemics, novel findings on dangerous pollutants in the environment, substances in food which prevent cancer, genes predisposing to disease or drugs promising to wipe them out, are reported regularly. Their actual relevance for human health depends crucially on the accumulation of evidence from studies, guided by the principles of epidemiology, that directly observe and evaluate what happens in human populations and groups.

These studies combine two features. They explore health and disease with the instruments of medical research, ranging from records of medical histories to measures of height, weight, blood pressure to a wide variety of diagnostic tests and procedures. At the same time they involve individuals living in society exposed to a multitude of influences, and they cannot be conducted in the isolated and fully controlled conditions of laboratory experiments. Their design, conduct and analysis require, instead, the methods of statistics and of social sciences such as demography, the quantitative study of human populations. Without a clear understanding of this composite nature of epidemiology and of its reasoning in terms of probability and statistics it is hard to appreciate the strengths and weaknesses of the scientific evidence relevant to medicine and public health that epidemiology keeps producing. It is not only among the general public that a woolly appreciation or even a frank misreading of epidemiology often surfaces, for instance in debates on risks or on the merit, real or imagined, of a disease treatment. In my experience the same may occur with journalists, members of ethics committees, health administrators, health policy makers and even with experts in disciplines other than epidemiology responsible for evaluating and funding research projects.

This *Very Short Introduction* is intended to give readers insight into what makes a difference between an epidemiological tale, be it about a magic pill or a fearful virus, and scientifically sound epidemiological evidence. The difference does not depend on how exciting or practically important the pill or the virus stories may be but solely on how well the epidemiological methods behind them have been applied. The methods and logic of epidemiology are a rather austere matter but I have attempted to give a flavour of the nature of the field with no mathematical symbols and formulas and only the simplest arithmetic. To set epidemiology into perspective its methods, logic and uses in medicine and public health are outlined against the backdrop of today's concerns for ethics and social justice in health.

My gratitude goes to the many colleagues and students, continuing sources of learning, that have made this book possible. My task has been facilitated by the cooperation and competence of the Oxford University Press staff. I owe personal thanks to Latha Menon for her sympathetic support and thoughtful advice throughout all phases of the book preparation and to Sharon Whelan who patiently revised my English.

List of illustrations

Chapter 1
What is epidemiology?

On 28 February 2003, the French Hospital of Hanoi, Vietnam, a private hospital of fewer than 60 beds, consulted the Hanoi office of the World Health Organization (WHO). A business traveller from Hong Kong had been hospitalized on 26 February for respiratory symptoms resembling influenza that had started three days before. The WHO medical officer, Dr Carlo Urbani, an infectious diseases epidemiologist and a previous member of Médecins sans Frontières, answered the call. Within days, in the course of which three more people fell ill with the same symptoms, he recognized the aggressiveness and the highly contagious nature of the disease. It looked like influenza but it wasn't. Early in March the first patient died, while similar cases started to show up in Hong Kong and elsewhere. Dr Urbani courageously persisted working in what he knew to be a highly hazardous environment. After launching a worldwide alert via the WHO surveillance network, he fell ill while travelling to Bangkok and died on 29 March. A run of new cases, some fatal, was now occurring not only among the staff of the French Hospital, but in Hong Kong, Taiwan, Singapore, mainland China, and Canada. Public health services were confronted with two related tasks: to build an emergency worldwide net of containment, while investigating the ways in which the contagion spread in order to pinpoint its origin and to discover how the responsible agent, most probably a micro-organism, was propagated. It took four months to identify the culprit of the new disease as a virus of the corona-virus family that had jumped to infect humans from wild small animals handled and consumed as food in the Guangdong province of China. By July 2003, the worldwide propagation of the virus, occurring essentially via infected air travellers, was blocked. The outbreak of the new disease, labelled SARS (Severe Acute Respiratory Syndrome), stopped at some 8,000 cases and 800 deaths. The toll would have been much heavier were it not for a remarkable international collaboration to control the spread of the virus through isolation of cases and control of wildlife markets. Epidemiology was at the heart of this effort, combining investigations in the populations hit by SARS with laboratory studies that provided the knowledge required for the disease-control interventions.

Epidemiology owes its name to 'epidemic', derived from the Greek *epi* (on) and *demos* (population). Epidemics like SARS that strike as unusual appearances of a disease in a population require immediate investigation, but essentially the same investigative approach applies to diseases in general, whether unusual in type or frequency or present all the time in a population in an 'endemic' form. In fact, the same methods are used to study normal physiological events such as reproduction and pregnancy, and physical and mental growth, in populations. Put concisely, *epidemiology is the study of health and disease in populations*.

The population aspect is the distinctive trait of epidemiology, while health and disease are investigated at other levels as well. In fact, when 'medicine' is referred to, without specification, one thinks spontaneously of clinical medicine that deals with health and disease in *individuals*. We may also imagine laboratory scientists carrying out biological experiments, the results of which may hopefully be translated into diagnostic or treatment innovations in clinical medicine. By contrast, the population dimension of health and disease, and with it epidemiology, is less prominent in the minds of most people. In the past, introduced to someone as an epidemiologist, I was not infrequently greeted with the remark

'I see you are a specialist treating skin diseases'. (Clearly the person thought of some fancy 'epidermology', alias dermatology. Now I introduce myself as a public health physician, which works much better.)

A flashback into history

Clear antecedents of contemporary epidemiology can be traced back more than 2,000 years. The writings of the great Greek physician Hippocrates (c. 470 to c. 400 BC) provide not only the first known descriptions, accurate and complete, of diseases such as tetanus, typhus, and phthisis (now tuberculosis of the lung), but also show an extraordinarily perceptive approach to the causes of diseases. Like a modern epidemiologist, Hippocrates does not confine his view of medicine and disease to his individual patients but sees health and disease as dependent on a broad context of environmental and lifestyle factors.

According to Hippocrates:

> Whoever wishes to investigate medicine properly should proceed thus: in the first place to consider the seasons of the year, and what effects each of them produces. Then the winds, the hot and the cold, especially such as are common to all countries, and then such as are peculiar to each locality. In the same manner, when one comes into a city to which he is a stranger, he should consider its situation, how it lies as to the winds and the rising of the sun; for its influence is not the same whether it lies to the north or to the south, to the rising or to the setting of the sun. One should consider most attentively the waters which the inhabitants use, whether they be marshy and soft, or hard and running from elevated and rocky situations, and then if saltish and unfit for cooking; and on the ground, whether it be naked and deficient in water, or wooded and well watered, and whether it lies in a hollow, confined situation, or it is elevated and cold; and the mode in which the inhabitants live, and what are their pursuits,

whether they are fond of drinking and eating to excess, and given to indolence, or are fond of exercise and labour.

Hippocrates, *On Airs, Waters and Places*

Many centuries would elapse, however, before epidemiology could move from perceptive observations and insights to a quantitative description and analysis of diseases in populations. The necessary premise was the revolution in science ushered in by Galileo Galilei (1564–1642), who for the first time systematically combined observation and measurement of natural phenomena with experiments designed to explore the underlying regulating laws, expressible in mathematical form (for example, the law of acceleration of falling bodies). The work of John Graunt (1620–74), a junior contemporary of Galilei, is a remarkable example of the general intellectual climate promoting accurate collection and quantitative analyses of data on natural phenomena. In his *Natural and Political Observations Upon the Bills of Mortality* of London, Graunt uses simple (by our standards) but rigorous mathematical methods to analyse mortality in the whole population, including comparisons between men and women and by type of diseases (acute or chronic). Later progress in epidemiology was made possible by two developments. First, the expansion in collection of data on the size and structure of populations by age and sex, and on vital events such as births and deaths; and second, advances in mathematical tools dealing with chance and probabilities, initially arising out of card and dice games, which were soon seen to be equally applicable to natural events like births and deaths.

By the early 19th century, most of the principles and ideas guiding today's epidemiology had already been established, as even a cursory look at the subsequent history shows.

In France, Pierre-Charles Alexandre Louis championed the fundamental principle that the effect of any potentially beneficial

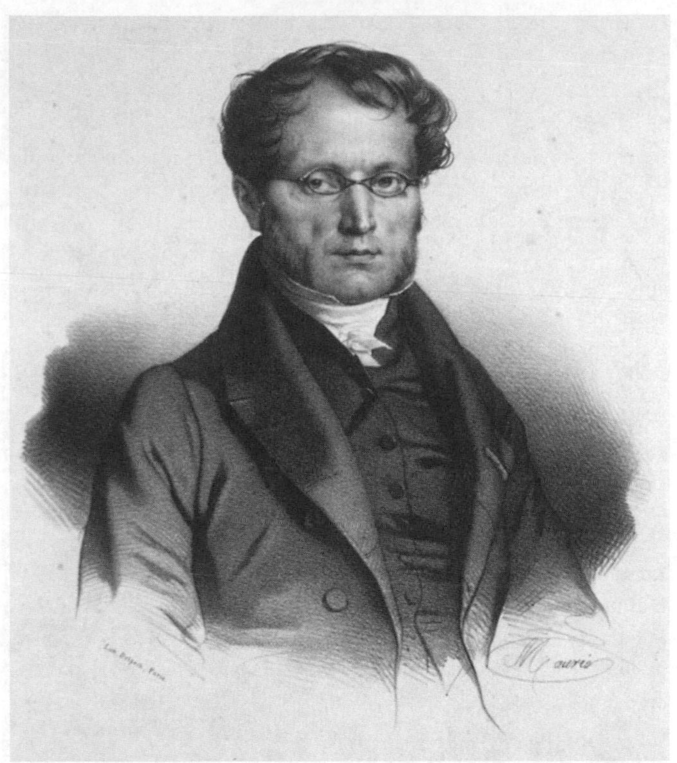

1a. Pierre-Charles Louis (1787–1872)

treatment, or of any toxic substance, can only be assessed by a comparison of closely similar subjects receiving and not receiving it. He used his 'numerical method' to produce statistical evidence that the then widespread practice of bloodletting was ineffective or even dangerous when contrasted with no treatment. In London, John Snow's research highlighted the idea that insightful epidemiological analyses of disease occurrence may produce enough knowledge to enable disease-prevention measures, even in ignorance of the specific agents at microscopic level. Snow conducted around the middle of the 19th century brilliant

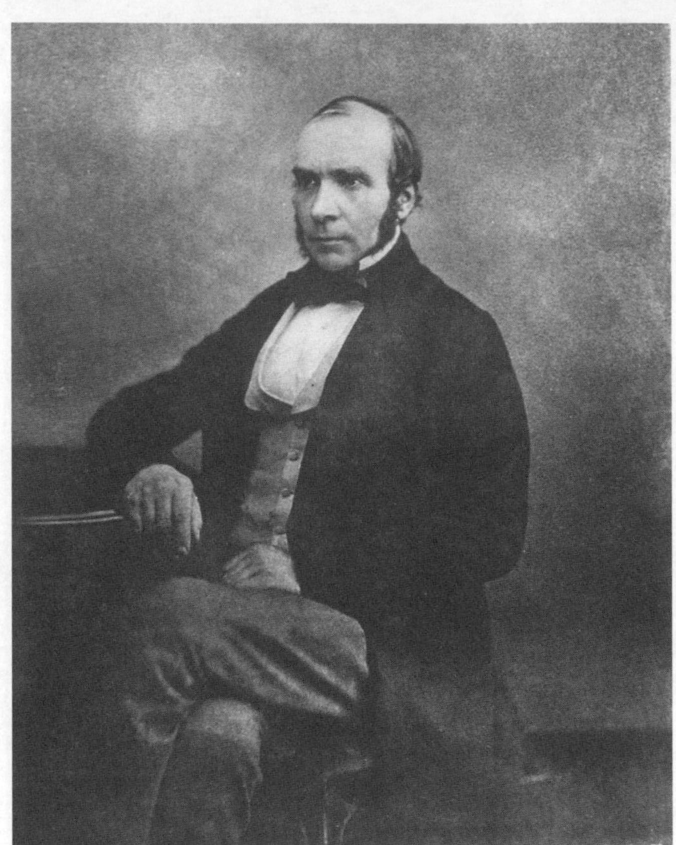

1b. John Snow (1813–1858)

investigations during cholera epidemics that led to the identification of drinking water polluted by sewage as the origin of the disease. This permitted the establishment of hygienic measures to prevent the pollution without knowing the specific noxious element the sewage was carrying. That factor, discovered some 20 years later, turned out to be a bacterium (*Vibrio cholerae*) excreted in the faeces by cholera patients and propagated via the sewage. In

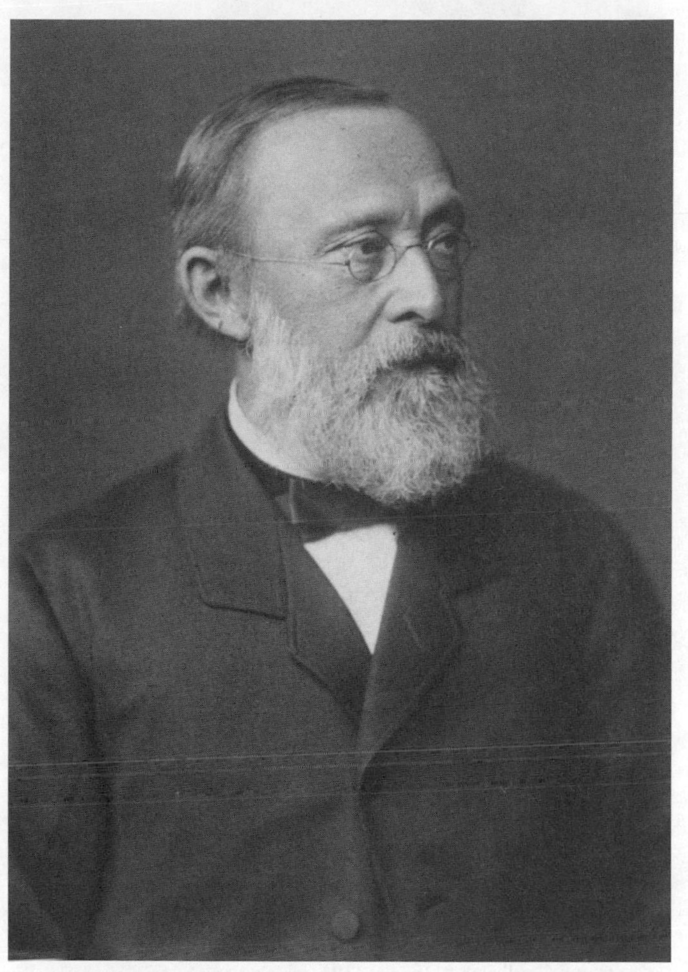

1c. **Rudolf Virchow (1821–1902)**

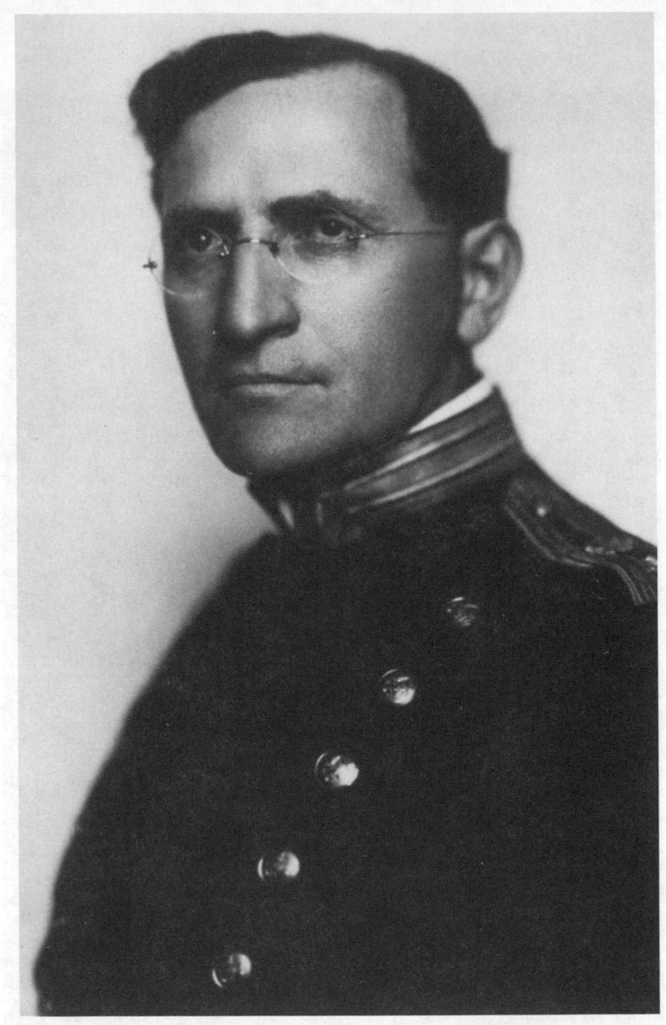

1d. Joseph Goldberger (1874–1929)

Germany, Rudolf Virchow forcefully promoted during the second part of the century the concept that medicine and public health are not only biological but also applied social sciences. Consistent with this inspiration, his studies ranged from pathology – he is acknowledged as the founder of cellular pathology – to epidemiological investigations backed by sociological enquiries. In the United States, the work of Joseph Goldberger demonstrated that epidemiology is equally well suited to identify infectious and non-infectious agents as possible origins of a disease. In the first three decades of the 20th century, he investigated pellagra, a serious neurological disease endemic in several areas of the Americas and Europe, reaching the conclusion that it was due not to an infectious agent, as most then believed, but to poor diet, deficient in a vitamin (later chemically identified and named vitamin PP). In the century spanning Louis to Goldberger, and in fact throughout its history up to the present day, epidemiology has received major support from advances in the contiguous field of statistics, a key ingredient of any epidemiological investigation.

Epidemiology today

Today's epidemiology developed particularly during the second half of the last century. By the end of World War II, it became apparent that in most economically advanced countries the burden of non-communicable diseases of unknown origin, such as cancer and cardiovascular disease, was becoming heavier than the load of communicable disease due to micro-organisms and largely controllable through hygiene measures, vaccinations, and treatment with antibiotics. These new circumstances provided a strong impetus for epidemiology to search for the unknown disease origins through new as well as established methods of research which soon came to be used beyond their initial scope in all areas of medicine and public health. This is reflected in the concept of epidemiology as the study of health and disease in populations:

> [Epidemiology is] the study of the occurrence and distribution of health-related states or events in specified populations, including the study of the determinants influencing such states, and the application of this knowledge to control the health problems.
>
> M. Porta, *A Dictionary of Epidemiology*

All aspects of health when studied at the level of population are the proper domain of epidemiology, which covers not only the description of how diseases and, more generally, health-related conditions occur in the population, but also the search for the factors, as a rule multiple, at their origin. This investigative activity is sustained by scientific curiosity but is firmly directed towards an applied objective: the prevention and treatment of disease and promotion of health. A fascinating and challenging feature of epidemiology is that it explores health and disease in connection with factors which, to take heart attacks as an example, span from the level of the molecule, say blood cholesterol, to the level of society, say loss of employment. This broad perspective makes epidemiology at the same time a biomedical and a social science. Epidemiological studies include both routine applications of epidemiological methods, for example in surveillance of communicable diseases or in monitoring of hospital admissions and discharges, and research investigations designed to generate new knowledge of general relevance. There may be overlaps and transitions between these two types of studies. When routine surveillance detects an outbreak of a previously unknown disease, like SARS, subsequent investigations produce factual knowledge that is at the same time useful for the local and practical purpose of controlling the disease and for the general scientific purpose of describing the new disease and the factors at its origin. Epidemiology fulfils the same diagnostic functions for the health of a community as a doctor's consultation does for the individual.

Within epidemiology a clear distinction must be made between *observational* and *intervention*, or *experimental*, studies. Experimental studies are dominant in the biomedical sciences. For example, scientists working in laboratories intervene all the time on whole animals, isolated organs, and cell cultures by administering drugs or toxic chemicals to study their effects. By contrast, within epidemiology, observational studies are by far the most common. Epidemiologists observe what happens in a group of people, record health-related events, ask questions, take measurements of the body or on blood specimens, but do not intervene actively in the lives or the environments of the subjects under study. Intervention studies, for example trials of new vaccines in the population, are an essential but smaller component of epidemiology, representing no more than one-fifth to one-tenth of all epidemiological studies in healthy populations. In populations of patients, however, trials of treatments, from drugs to surgery, are most common. All kinds of studies, whether routine or for research, observational or experimental, stand with their own particularities on the common basis of the epidemiological principles outlined in this volume.

Five major areas within epidemiology

1. *Descriptive epidemiology*: describes health and disease and their trends over time in specific populations.
2. *Aetiological epidemiology*: searches for hazardous or beneficial factors influencing health conditions (e.g. toxic pollutants, inappropriate diet, deadly micro-organisms; beneficial diets, behavioural habits to improve fitness).
3. *Evaluative epidemiology*: evaluates the effects of preventive interventions; quantitatively estimates risks of specific diseases for persons exposed to hazardous factors.
4. *Health services epidemiology*: describes and analyses the work of health services.
5. *Clinical epidemiology*: describes the natural course of a disease in a patient population and evaluates the effects of diagnostic procedures and of treatments.

Chapter 2
Measuring health and disease

> Health is a state of complete physical, mental and social well-being and not merely the absence of disease or infirmity.
>
> Constitution of the World Health Organization, 7 April 1948

One may wonder whether the founding fathers, who in the aftermath of World War II inscribed the definition of health in the World Health Organization (WHO) constitution, unconsciously had in mind happiness rather than health, although even happiness, a changing and intermittent human experience, cannot be accurately described as a heavenly and lasting state of perfect well-being. Abstract as it is, the WHO definition does have the merit of stressing the relevance of the psychological and social dimensions, beyond those purely physiological, of health and disease (social aspects incorporated in a recent WHO classification of disabilities and social determinants of health have been a central theme for the organization in recent years). Even today, for the majority of humankind the basic objective of achieving absence of disease or infirmity, as far as may be possible by current preventive and therapeutic means, remains unattainable, nor is it clear when it may be attained. Hence measuring health starting from its negative, the presence of disease, is not only technically easier but also makes practical sense.

Defining disease

For the purpose of epidemiological study, a disease can be defined either by creating a definition and regarding as cases the subjects that fit it or by accepting as cases those subjects that have been so diagnosed by a doctor. In an epidemiological survey of diabetes it may be decided that a study team directly examines a fraction of all adults in a town and regards as diabetic those people who satisfy a pre-fixed set of diagnostic criteria. Alternatively, and much more simply, one can accept as cases the people declared to be diabetic by doctors in the general practices and hospitals of the town. Actually the two approaches may to some extent overlap. When carrying out a direct survey, the study team will in fact come across some subjects already known to be diabetic and for whom further tests may be deemed unnecessary. Accepting existing diagnoses may, however, result in data perturbed by differences in disease definition and diagnostic practice between doctors in the area, a drawback not shared by a direct full-blown epidemiological survey carried out with a fixed definition and uniform procedures. An intermediate solution between a more reliable but cumbersome survey and a simpler but less reliable face-value acceptance of existing diagnoses may consist of confirming or rejecting the diagnosis only after thoroughly reviewing the medical records in the physician and hospital files. Still, this procedure would not capture, as an epidemiological survey would, the not infrequent cases of diabetes present in the population that do not show up in the files because those affected have no symptoms. Any of these approaches to the definition of diabetes and case identification may be employed to produce figures on the frequency of diabetes in a country, a region, or a particular group of people.

To complicate matters, many disease definitions have changed and continue to change, sometimes even in a major way, with advances in biological and medical knowledge. In the case of diabetes, the threshold levels for sugar in the blood that define diabetes were modified ten years ago taking into account the results of several studies showing that levels previously regarded as 'normal' and safe were in fact associated with an increased frequency of complications. For heart attacks, the different types of myocardial infarction are currently redefined including among the criteria the detection in the blood of some hitherto unmeasurable proteins released by the damaged heart cells. Epidemiology itself may contribute to defining or redefining diseases. Rather than committing himself to a disease definition, the epidemiologist may simply measure individual symptoms such as insomnia, headache, fatigue, tremors, or nausea to see whether they occur jointly, forming a 'syndrome' (a cluster of symptoms) in individuals with special personal traits or in particular settings. This paves the way to the investigation of the physiological mechanisms, the external circumstances, and the progress in time of the syndrome; once these elements become clear, the definition of a new disease or a special form of a disease already known may be consolidated.

Defining and diagnosing diabetes

Diabetes 'mellitus' (honey-sweet) takes its name from the loss of sugar that makes urine sweet. It occurs in two forms. Type 1, or juvenile, diabetes starts most commonly before the age of 30, while type 2, or adult, diabetes mostly begins after the age of 30. Both types, which differ in their underlying lesions and response to treatment, have in common an impairment of the metabolism of sugars leading to abnormal levels of glucose in the blood. Among the consequences are the passage of glucose in the urine and a high level of glucose in the body tissues, inducing a series of complications in the cardiovascular and nervous systems. It is the progression of these complications that makes diabetes a potentially very serious disease.

The diagnosis of diabetes may be suspected by the presence of symptoms such as excessive urination and thirst, recurrent infections, and unexplained weight loss (particularly in type 1, or from previous overweight in type 2). It becomes established if the level of glucose in plasma (the liquid fraction of blood) in a person fasting for 8 to 12 hours equals or exceeds 126 milligrams per decilitre. Many diabetes cases, particularly of type 2, present no symptoms for several years and are recognized only through a routine blood test done for other reasons: in this situation, the diagnosis is regarded as established only if a repeated blood test in a fasting condition confirms the result of the first.

Within an epidemiological survey carried out for research purposes, the best single diagnostic tool is to have the fasting subjects drink a concentrated solution of 75 grams of glucose and measure the glucose plasma level after 2 hours. A level of 200 milligrams per decilitre or above is diagnostic for diabetes, while values between 140 and 199 milligrams indicate an impaired regulation of glucose, a condition that increases the likelihood of developing diabetes.

Reference disease definitions are found in medical textbooks and collections of definitions have been developed, the best known and most widely used being the International Classification of Diseases and Related Health Problems (abridged as ICD) of the World Health Organization. As the name indicates, ICD is not a mere collection of disease definitions but a 'nosological' (from the Greek *nosos*, disease) system of ordering and grouping diseases. The grouping scheme has evolved out of that proposed in the early phases of international discussions on disease classification some 150 years ago. It reflects the same compromise between two main criteria of classification, one based on the site of the disease in the body and one based on the nature and origin of the disease. It covers five broad areas: communicable diseases of infectious origin; constitutional or general diseases (blood diseases, metabolic diseases like diabetes, cancers, mental disorders); diseases of specific organs or systems (cardiovascular, digestive, etc.); diseases related to pregnancy, birth, and development;

diseases arising from injuries and poisons. The first edition of the ICD was adopted in 1900 during an international conference in Paris at which 26 countries were represented. Revisions took place at 10-yearly intervals, and in 1948 the newly established World Health Organization took charge of the 6th revision and became responsible for all subsequent developments. Currently the 10th revision (ICD-10), which has been updated annually since 1996 rather than being completely revised, is in use.

ICD-10 is organized into 22 disease categories, each being denoted by a three-character code composed of one letter and two numbers. The different types of diabetes mellitus have codes E10 to E14 and are included in category IV, 'Endocrine, nutritional, and metabolic diseases'. Myocardial infarction is coded I21, within the category IX, 'Diseases of the circulatory system'; a fourth digit, to be used optionally, makes it possible to specify the part of the heart wall affected by the infarction. The three-character code is used in all countries that keep some system of health statistics to code the disease regarded as the cause of death. In many countries, it is also used in its standard form or with extensions and modifications for coding diagnoses in hospital discharge or other health services' records. Tables allowing conversion of codes between different versions of ICD have been developed. Death is an unequivocal event and mortality statistics are an established yardstick for the description of the health conditions of a population.

Causes of death, as recorded in death certificates that use ICD-10, are subject to the problems of diagnosis already mentioned and require translating a doctor's diagnosis into ICD codes. The internationally adopted death certificate provides a simple standard format to facilitate the task of the doctor in identifying the 'underlying' cause of death among the several ailments that may affect a patient. A full set of rules, today often in computerized form, is then available to the coders who have to convert the death certificate information into ICD codes. Notwithstanding these procedures, the accuracy of coded causes of death is still imperfect and variable even in developed countries. In developing countries, where more than three quarters of the world population live and die, reaching a minimally acceptable level of accuracy in the absence of adequate medical services may demand a 'verbal autopsy', i.e. a systematic retrospective enquiry of family members about the symptoms of illness prior to death. These limitations need to be kept in mind when dealing with mortality statistics, and more generally with statistics based on disease diagnoses. Yet as the British medical statistician Major Greenwood remarked: 'The scientific purist, who will wait for medical statistics until they are nosologically exact, is no wiser than Horace's rustic waiting for the river to flow away.'

Measuring disease

Three elements are always needed to measure the occurrence of a disease in a population or in a group within the population: the number of cases of the disease, the number of people in the population, and an indication of time. The finding that in the adult (age 15 and over) male population of Flower City, 5,875 cases of type 2 diabetes mellitus have been observed has a very different significance in a male population of Flower City of 10,000 than in 100,000 or 1,000,000 men. To make this relation explicit, a first measure of occurrence can be computed, the '*prevalence proportion*' or simply '*prevalence*':

$$prevalence\ proportion = \frac{number\ of\ diseased\ persons}{number\ of\ persons\ in\ the\ population}$$

If the number of persons (men) in the population is actually 45,193, the prevalence proportion is: 5,875 / 45,193 = 0.13. In percentage form, 13% of all adult males in Flower City are diabetic. Now, or some time in the past? If the count was made in 1908 or 1921, it may be only of historical interest; if in a recent year, it is of current interest and carries practical implications. The point in time at which the census of the cases and of the population was taken needs to be specified, say 1 January 2008. This completes our measure and makes it unambiguous as an instant picture of diabetes in the Flower City male population. The information is useful, for instance, for the planning of health services. In general prevalence figures for all health conditions and in the different sections of the population, males and females, young or old, are required to plan an adequate provision of health services for diagnosis and treatment. It takes just a little reflection to realize that the prevalence of diabetes reflects in fact the balance between two opposite processes: the appearance of new cases and the disappearance of existing cases who die (or if they were completely cured, which happens for some diseases, such as pneumonia, but not for established diabetes). Both processes develop in time, hence time should now be taken not as a simple indication of the point at

Probability and risk

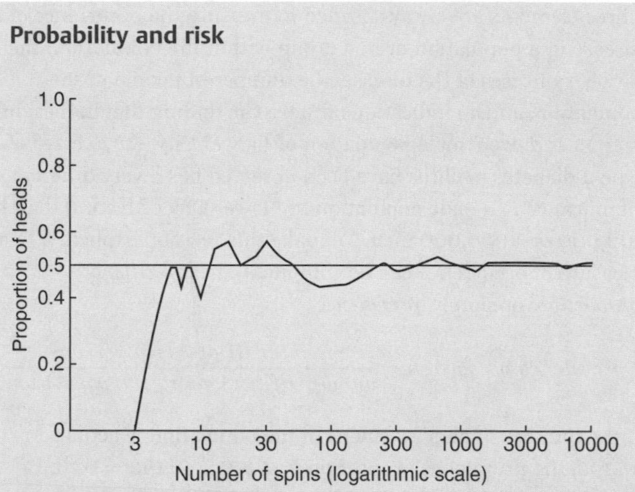

2. The proportions of heads in a sequence of spins of a coin

Before a soccer match, the referee tosses a coin to assign 'at random' a side to each team in the playing field. The procedure is fair to the two teams by assuming that a perfect coin will not fall preferentially on heads or tails. The results of an experiment in which the results of 10,000 tosses were recorded show that this is a tenable assumption. As portrayed in the figure, the proportion of heads varies widely when the number of spins is small, but the variation decreases and the proportion becomes gradually more stable as the number of tosses increases. The coin does not compensate in some mysterious way for any series of consecutive heads that may have occurred with an equal number of tails: simply, any imbalance between heads and tails will be diluted as the number of tosses increases and the value of the proportion will tend to stabilize more and more closely around the value 0.50 (or if you prefer 50%). This value – hypothetical, as in principle the series of tosses should carry on indefinitely – can be taken as the probability of a head. In general, '*the probability of an event is the proportion of occasions the event occurs in an indefinitely long series of occasions*'. Being a proportion, it ranges between zero and one, or, in percentages, from 0 to 100%.

The notion of risk relates probability to time. '*Risk is the probability of an event in a specified interval of time*', for instance of breaking a leg within the next five years. Risk should not be confused, as often happens in common parlance, with a *risk factor*, also called *hazard*, entailing the risk of some harmful effect: for fractures of the leg bones, skiing is a risk factor. As here defined, risk is simply the probability of any effect, harmful or beneficial, for example recovery from a disease.

which the measurement was made (as for prevalence) but as time intervals within which new cases and deaths occur.

Disease risk and disease incidence rates

The risk of a disease is the probability that a person becomes diseased during the time of observation:

$$risk = \frac{number\ of\ persons\ who\ become\ diseased\ during\ a\ time\ period}{number\ of\ persons\ at\ the\ beginning\ of\ time\ period}$$

If in the population of Flower City (no. 45,193), 226 new cases of diabetes were diagnosed in the period between 1 January and 31 December 2008, the risk is 226/45,193 = 0.005 or 5.0 per 1,000 persons. This simple measure provides an estimate of the risk for a male living in Flower City to become diabetic if the population of the town is 'closed', with no individuals entering or leaving for whatever reason. Clearly a real natural population is never closed: people die, people move out and come in. Even in an artificially formed population such as a group of people identified for long-term follow-up and study of health, with no further entries permitted into the group, there will be deaths and some people will inevitably become untraceable. In short, risk seems a too crude measure in most circumstances except when the time interval of observation is so short, not a year but a week or a day, that entries into and exits from the population are minimal and can be ignored.

These shortcomings are not shared by a related measure of disease occurrence, the *incidence rate*, which is of general use but requires a more subtle formulation and the availability of more detailed data than just the number of people present at the beginning of the time of observation and the number of subjects who have developed diabetes by the end of that time. The incidence rate can be regarded as the probability of developing the disease in a time interval so tiny, just an instant, that no two events (death, arrival of an immigrant, new case of a disease, etc.) can take place within it. It is an instantaneous rate of occurrence, called *instantaneous death rate* when the event is death (the expressive term *force of mortality* is also used) and *instantaneous morbidity rate* when the event is the occurrence of a new case of a disease. The incidence rate can be derived as:

$$incidence\ rate = \frac{number\ of\ persons\ who\ become\ diseased\ while\ observed}{sum\ of\ individual\ observation\ times\ of\ all\ persons}$$

The 'observation period' of a person is the length of time from the start of the observation to the moment he/she develops the disease or dies or is no longer under observation because he/she is lost from sight or the study has come to an end. The individual times of observation are summed and form the denominator of the rate. If, while the population of Flower City was observed during the 365 days between 1 January and 31 December 2008, a subject has migrated out on 31 March, after 90 days, he/she should be counted not as one person but only as 90/365 = 0.25 person-years; if somebody died on 29 August, he/she should be counted for 241/365 = 0.66 person-years. The measurement unit *person-year* captures the key concept that each person should count not as one but as an amount equal to the time he or she has been actually exposed to the risk of developing the disease. For the male population of Flower City, the incidence rate of diabetes, properly calculated in this way, turned out to be 5.2 per 1,000 person-years, or – in a less accurate but often-used expression – 5.2 per 1,000 per year. In plain words, some 5 men out of 1,000 become diabetic every year. Time is usually and arbitrarily specified as year, but week or even day may be more convenient when dealing with acute outbreaks of diseases such as influenza or SARS. In these instances, the measurement unit becomes *person-week* or *person-day*.

Intuitively, the incidence rate must have a positive relation to the prevalence proportion. More new cases of diabetes feed a higher prevalence of diabetes in the population if the average duration of the disease, which depends on how soon death intervenes after the disease onset, does not change in time. For the Flower City male population, in stable conditions, it is sufficient to multiply the incidence rate of 5.2 per 1,000 person-years by an average duration of diabetes of roughly 25 years to obtain the prevalence of 13% described before.

A rate, in epidemiology as in all sciences, is a measure incorporating time as the reference. A rate of interest is how much you gain per year out of a capital, a rate of progression in space or velocity (speed) is how long a distance you cover in one minute or one hour. The term 'rate' should be confined to this use and not extended generically to other types of ratios. If you hear of 'prevalence rate', it is a wrong expression simply meaning prevalence proportion. *Crude rates* of incidence or mortality refer to a whole population, while *specific rates*, e.g. age-specific or sex-specific, refer to population subgroups defined by age or by sex.

The arithmetic of incidence rate

The incidence rate is a fundamental measure in epidemiology and demography. When computed for a healthy population, it expresses the probability of new cases of a disease per unit of time. When referring to a population of diseased persons, it expresses the probability of dying, or of recovering, per unit of time.

Imagine that a mini-population of 10 people has been observed for a winter trimester, i.e. 13 weeks after 1 January 2000, in a medical practice. Two new cases of influenza have been diagnosed, Blondine at week 6 and Frank at week 10, giving a risk of influenza of 2/10 = 0.2, or 20% in the trimester. Andrew, a foreign traveller, has come under observation on week 2 and left on week 4; George moved out for his job on week 9; and Ian unfortunately died in an accident in week 11. For simplicity, all events (arrival, departure, death, diagnosis of influenza) are regarded as occurring at the mid-point of a week. Andrew was observed for only 2 weeks, hence his time at risk of developing influenza is 2 weeks; Blondine developed influenza during the 6th week, hence her time at risk is 5.5 weeks, because the subsequent time of observation until week 13 no longer presents risk of influenza from the same strain of virus. The weeks at risk for Andrew, Blondine, and all the others are shown in the third column of the table.

	Weeks of observation	Influenza diagnosed at week	Weeks at risk
Andrew	2	-	2
Blondine	13	6th	5.5
Charles	13	-	13
Diana	13	-	13
Eve	13	-	13
Frank	13	10th	9.5
George	8.5	-	8.5
Helen	13	-	13
Ian	10.5	-	10.5
Jenny	13	-	13

The incidence rate can now be computed as 2 / (2 + 5.5 + 13 + … 10.5 + 13) = 2/101 = 0.0198 per person-week or 1.98 per 100 person-weeks. 2 persons out of every 100 falling ill in the short interval of one week is a high rate. Ostensibly, in 52 weeks (a year) 104 persons (2 × 52), out of a total of 100 would fall ill, a plainly absurd result! In fact, a correct calculation, which involves more than simple arithmetic, would show that if this rate had continued for the whole year (which by good fortune does not usually happen with seasonal influenza), only 3 or perhaps 4 of the 10 persons in our mini-population would have escaped it.

Chapter 3
Searching for the causes of disease

Disease causes and exposures

We use the word 'cause' frequently in everyday parlance. The concept seems intuitively simple, yet it proves logically problematic and has been subject to continuous debate ever since Greek philosophers, in particular Aristotle, started to define it in the 5th century BC. Causes of disease do not escape this difficulty. When a few hours after a club dinner several members fall sick with gastroenteritis, what is the cause? The dinner, without which the intestinal trouble would have not occurred? The 'tiramisu' dessert, as only those who ate it fell sick? The bacterium *Staphylococcus aureus* which, as a subsequent laboratory investigation showed, had found its way into the 'tiramisu' through a lapse in hygiene in the kitchen? The toxin produced by the bacterium that attacks the cells of the intestinal lining? The biologically active part of the toxin molecule that binds to some molecules of the cell membrane? It could be tempting to take the latter as the ultimate, hence 'real', cause, but our understanding of the world would fast dissolve if only relationships between molecules could qualify as causal. For instance, it would be impossible to describe and analyse the circulation of the blood in terms of individual molecules. It is only when molecules join to form higher-order, complex structures such as blood cells, arteries, veins, the heart muscle, that new properties emerge permitting explanation of the working of the circulatory system. In fact, in our club dinner example each factor, from the dinner itself to the active part of the molecule, can be regarded legitimately, at a different level of observation and detail, as a cause. Without *any one* of them there would have been no gastroenteritis. In general, we can consider as a cause a factor without which an effect, adverse such as disease or favourable like the protection against it, would not have happened.

Most of the epidemiologist's investigative work consists in trying to identify the 'factors without which' a disease would or would not arise. In terms of the actual disease measurements introduced in Chapter 2, this means to identify factors of any nature – social, biological, chemical, physical – whose presence can be shown to be constantly associated with an increase or a decrease in a disease incidence rate or risk. There are scores of candidates for this role, from stress at work to inherited genes, from fatty foods to physical exercise, from drugs to air pollutants. They can all be designated with the generic label of *factor* or (in epidemiological jargon) *exposure*, neutral enough not to prejudice whether the candidate will in the end come out as a cause of disease or not.

Comparing rates and risks while minimizing biases

The usually long research journey to show that a factor is a cause of disease starts by comparing incidence rates or risks between different groups of people. Noting that the rate of occurrence of type 2 diabetes is higher in a group of overweight people observed for several years than in people of normal weight suggests that excessive weight may be among the determinants of diabetes. Before this suggestion can be transformed into conclusive evidence, two conditions need to be fulfilled: (1) demonstrating that there is an association between the exposure, overweight, and diabetes incidence, the theme of this chapter; (2) interpreting that association as causal in nature, discussed in Chapter 4.

Overweight people may differ from people of normal weight in many respects: gender, age, diet, amount of physical exercise, and any of these, rather than excess weight itself, may be responsible for the increase in the rate of onset of diabetes. As a first step to tackling this problem, we can exclude some of the possible interfering factors by restricting our study to normal and overweight people belonging to only one gender and age range, say males aged 40 to 59 in Flower City. Being overweight is defined as having a body mass index (BMI) of more than 25. BMI gauges weight in relation to a person's height (it is computed as the ratio of weight divided by the square of height): a BMI in the range 19 to 25 is regarded as normal. People with a BMI higher than 25 are considered overweight, and within this category those with a BMI over 30 are classified as obese. The approach of removing possible interfering factors by confining the study to only some categories of people soon reaches its limit. Restricting further the study to, say, sedentary people eating a specific type of diet will not only drastically reduce the number of subjects available for investigation but, worse, it may also make its results inapplicable to the population in general. A better, and in fact the most commonly employed, method consists in acquiring and recording for each subject information on factors such as diet and physical exercise so that at the time of data analysis the comparison between normal and overweight people can be made not overall but first within subgroups (so-called 'strata') with the same type of diet and level of physical activity, and then summarized in an overall 'adjusted' comparison, freed of the influence of these factors.

According to the study design just mentioned, a cohort of 3,000 volunteer males, aged 40 to 59, free of diabetes and resident in Flower City, has been recruited and followed up for one year, recording the new cases of type 2 diabetes. At recruitment, 1,980 subjects turned out to have a normal weight, while 1,020 were overweight. During the one-year follow-up, 15 new cases of diabetes and 45 deaths (from any cause) were recorded among the former, and 23 cases of diabetes and 49 deaths among the latter.

Results of a one-year observation of a cohort of 3,000 men in Flower City

Weight – Age	Number	Per cent	No. deaths	No. cases	Person-years	Rate
NORMAL WEIGHT						
40–49	1,173	59%	20	6	1,160	5.2
50–59	807	41%	25	9	790	11.4
40–59	1,980	100%	45	15	1,950	7.7
OVER WEIGHT						
40–49	198	19%	8	2	193	10.4
50–59	822	81%	41	21	791	26.5
40–59	1,020	100%	49	23	984	23.4

The person-years derive from assuming that subjects dying or becoming new cases of diabetes remained at risk of such events on average for one half of the year of observation. Hence the person-years for people of normal weight aged 40–49 are computed as: $1{,}173 - (20 + 6)/2 = 1{,}160$, and the person-years for the other groups are derived in the same way.

Among the normal weight subjects, the 15 cases of diabetes occurred out of 1,950 person-years at risk of developing the disease, an incidence rate of 7.7 per 1,000 person-years. For the overweight subjects, the 23 cases occurred out of 984 person-years, an incidence rate of 23.4 per 1,000 person-years. It is, however, disturbing to realize that enrolling only men aged 40 to 59, rather than all adult males, has not sufficed to remove the possible influence of age. The percentage of older people, aged 50–59, who are overweight is in fact about double (81%) the percentage (41%) who are normal weight, and this might be the real reason for the higher rate of new cases of diabetes, as it is well established that diabetes incidence increases with age. To remove the influence of age, we need to compare the rates between two groups having each the same composition by age, the simplest being 50% of people aged 40–49 and 50% of people aged 50–59. If these 'standard', i.e. fixed, percentages apply, the rates of 5.2 and 11.4 for the two age subgroups among the normal-weight people would each have an equal importance (or, technically, have the same 'weight') and their average rate would simply be $(5.2 + 11.4)/2 = 8.3$. Similarly for the overweight people, the average rate would be $(10.4 + 26.5)/2 = 18.5$. These two rates are *age-adjusted* by a standardization procedure: they still differ $(18.5 - 8.3 = 10.2)$ but materially less than the two overall, or crude, rates $(23.4 - 8.3 = 15.1)$.

After removing the influence of age, a difference remains that may indeed reflect an effect of weight or, annoyingly, of other potentially interfering factors like amount of exercise or diet. In fact, what is generally done in epidemiological studies is to adjust the rates not only for a single factor like age but for all interfering factors – called confounders or confounding factors – known to be capable of inducing a difference in rates. A host of statistical methods, much more complex than the simple standardization procedure just outlined, are currently available in computer software packages for implementing simultaneous adjustment for multiple confounders. The most often used appear in scientific papers under such names as *Cox's regression* (or *proportional hazard regression*) and *Poisson regression* for adjusting rates and *logistic regression* for adjusting risks. Regression has nothing to do with decadence but is a general term for a wide family of statistical methods analysing the dependency of one variable, for example an incidence rate, on several other variables such as gender, age, diet, and so on. (The name arises from one of the first uses of the method. When studying the relation between the heights of fathers and sons it was found that the sons of fathers taller than the mean tended to be on average less tall than the fathers, i.e. their stature tended to 'regress' towards the mean, the same regression occurring for sons of fathers shorter than the mean.)

Adjusting for confounders aims at eliminating the error that can arise by attributing to one factor, overweight, a difference in rates that may in fact be due to one or more other factors (the *confounders*). This is, however, only one source of possible error, two other main sources arising from the selection of people included in a study and from the methods of observing them. As seen, the Flower City cohort was composed of 3,000 male volunteers. If more overweight (but not normal weight) people of lower socio-economic classes had tended to volunteer for the study than overweight people of higher socio-economic classes, the higher rate of diabetes among the overweight subjects could reflect an effect of the less healthy diet of the lower classes rather than of obesity. This *selection bias* could go unrecognized and lead to a wrong interpretation of the study results if information on socio-economic conditions, which may not be simple to fully capture, would not have been collected on all subjects. An *observation bias* would, on the other hand, be introduced if, for example, overweight people had been kept under closer surveillance, because of their very condition, than normal-weight people. This may have made it more likely that new cases of diabetes would be detected among the overweight than among the normal-weight men. In sum, three types of potential distortions loom over any observational study in epidemiology: (a) bias from uncontrolled or inadequately controlled (through adjustment methods) confounders; (b) bias from selection of subjects; and (c) bias from observation of subjects and collection of information. Bias is synonymous with systematic or constant error, the most important and difficult to neutralize or at least to take into account in observational studies. In addition chance errors are always present.

Ruling out chance

For the Flower City cohort, we are told by the investigators that no other confounders than age and no selection and observation biases have proved relevant, hence only excess weight remains as a candidate for the observed association with the rates of diabetes. Yet how can one be reasonably sure that the difference between the age-adjusted incidence rates of diabetes (18.5 and 8.3) has not arisen purely by chance? Looking at the table of results, we see that in the age group 50–59 the number of person-years among normal-weight and overweight people happens to be rather large and essentially the same (790 and 791). We can take advantage of this circumstance and argue that if weight had no effect we would expect that, the person-years being the same, the number of new cases of diabetes would also be the same among normal and overweight people in the age group 50–59. Instead, there are 9 cases among people of normal weight and 21 among overweight subjects, a rather large divergence with respect to the expectation of an equal number of $(21 + 9)/2 = 15$. Even large divergences can, however, occur just by chance and the relevant question is: how often? We may exactly mimic our diabetes study by taking a coin, throwing it 30 times, noting the number of heads and tails, and repeating the experiment several times. The expectation is that there will be an equal number of heads and tails (15) in each experiment, as there should have been an equal number of diabetes cases (15) among normal and overweight people. The divergence from this expectation in the successive experiments, each consisting of 30 throws, will tell how likely or unlikely is a chance deviation as large as the one observed (21 and 9). Here are the results of a small series of 20 experiments that I did, before becoming tired:

Head	Tail	Head	Tail	Head	Tail	Head	Tail
11	19	14	16	11	19	15	15
15	15	14	16	11	19	17	13
13	17	16	14	12	18	**7**	**23**
11	19	13	17	18	12	14	16
11	19	14	16	16	14	15	15

One experiment out of 20 (5%) gave a result of 7 to 23 (in bold), a chance divergence from expectation larger than the one (21 to 9) observed in the data on diabetes. In 19 out of 20 experiments (95%), the divergence was instead less than 21 to 9. 95% is not 100%, but it is reasonably close to it, and on this basis we may be prepared to conclude that having observed in our study (which exactly mimics the head and tail experiments), 21 cases of diabetes among the overweight and 9 among the normal-weight people, the hypothesis that there is no real difference in rates can now be rejected. In statistical jargon, we have performed a *significance test* on the rate difference and we are prepared to say that 'the observed difference is statistically significant at the

5% level'. This implies that if we keep to this way of proceeding on similar occasions we are bound to be wrong only in 5% of them. Unfortunately, nobody can tell whether this may be one of those five occasions when we may 'reasonably' reach the wrong conclusion!

Significance tests and confidence limits

Carrying out head-and-tail experiments is a useful device to illustrate empirically the basis of a significance test, but exact calculations can be and are made every day based on probability theory. In the case of two alternative and mutually exclusive events, such as heads and tails, male and female, alive or dead, the binomial probability distribution permits exact calculations of how often an event that has a probability π of occurrence will in fact happen in n trials, for example how often in families of $n = 2$ children there will be 0 boys and 2 girls, 1 boy and 1 girl, and 2 boys and 0 girls. We assume (although it may not be strictly so in nature) that the successive births are independent in respect to sex determination and that the probability π of a male birth is ½, the same as the probability of a female birth. Hence the probability of 2 girls and 0 boys will be $½ \times ½ = ¼$ or 0.25, which is the probability of 2 boys and 0 girls as well. Moreover, any of the combinations of 1 boy and 1 girl will have a probability of $½ \times ½ = ¼$; as there are two possible combinations one with boy first girl second and the other with girl first, their total probability will be $2 \times ¼ = ½$ or 0.5. The three possible offspring cover all possibilities hence their probabilities must add up to 1, as they in fact do: $0.25 + 0.5 + 0.25 = 1$. In a similar way, probabilities can be derived for binomial distributions with other values of n and π.

In Figure 3, the height of the bars measures the probability of finding 0, 1, 2, 3, ... 30 overweight cases of diabetes out of $n = 30$ cases, when the probability π of a case being normal or overweight is ½ or 0.5. The numerical values of the probabilities are marked on

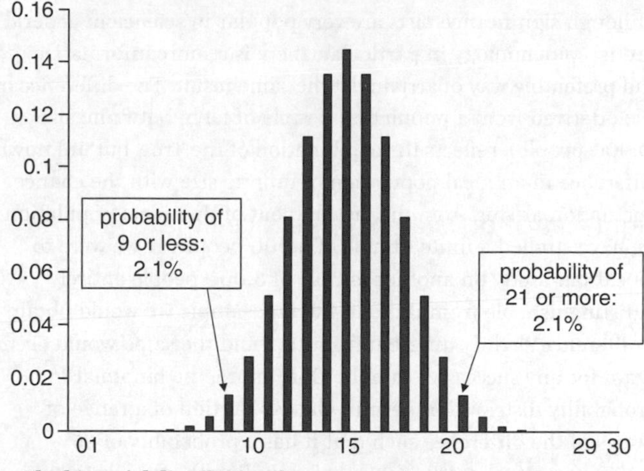

3. The binomial distribution for $\pi = 0.5$ and n = 30

the vertical axis and they add up to 1, i.e. certainty, as the 30 different outcomes exhaust all the possibilities. The sum of the probabilities (bars) in the right tail of the distribution for 21 or more overweight diabetes cases is 0.021 or 2.1%, and the symmetrical sum in the left tail, corresponding to 9 or fewer overweight diabetes cases, is also 2.1%. They add up to 4.2%, which confirms the finding of our mini-series of head-and-tail experiments. There is a probability of 4.2%, i.e. of less than 5% (routinely indicated as $p < 0.05$ or $P < 0.05$), that under the hypothesis called *null hypothesis* – of no difference in the incidence rate of diabetes between normal and overweight people – a result as extreme as 21 or more overweight cases would be observed. The same conclusion would have been reached if instead of focusing only on the people in the age bracket 50–59, we had performed our test of statistical significance on the age-adjusted rates of 18.5 and 8.3 that summarize the experience of the whole cohort of 3,000 men: their difference of 10.2 – the most relevant to test – turns out to be also statistically significant with probability $p < 0.05$.

Although significance tests are very popular in science in general and in epidemiology in particular, there is a more informative and preferable way of arriving at the same result. The difference of 10.2, derived from a population sample of large but finite size (3,000 people), reflects the combination of the 'true' but unknown difference in an ideal population of infinite size with the chance fluctuation arising from the fact that out of that ideal population we have studied a finite sample of 3,000 people. If we were to repeat our study on another sample of 3,000 people entirely indistinguishable from those in the first sample we would obtain a difference slightly different from 10.2 and the same would occur again for any successive sample. Once more, the binomial probability distribution permits the exploration of a range of values of the difference such that it has a probability of 95% (or if one prefers, 90% or 99%) of including the true unknown difference. For our case, these values are 2.0 and 18.3, a rather large range. We can summarize by saying that the *point estimate* of the true unknown difference is 10.2, with *95% confidence limits* (or with a *95% confidence interval*) of 2.0 and 18.3. In simple terms, the confidence interval expresses the range of values within which the true difference has a certain probability of being included. If there was no real difference, the range would include the value zero, i.e. it would, for instance, range from −3.2 to 11.5. The confidence interval is much more informative than a statistical significance test, and is therefore a much better way of assessing the role of chance. It not only tells us, like the significance test, that a difference is unlikely to have arisen by chance (if the null hypothesis were true), but provides information on the range of plausible values of that difference. Because the range does not provide a certainty but only specifies a probability that the true difference lies within it, it may be in error in the same way as a significance test. Computing 95% confidence limits and stating that the true difference lies between them will prove wrong on 5% of the occasions, but nobody can tell whether our diabetes study is one of these.

the rotten
crummy
LUCK !
only 1 in 1000
wrong
and that one
is MY
1 billion $
study !!!

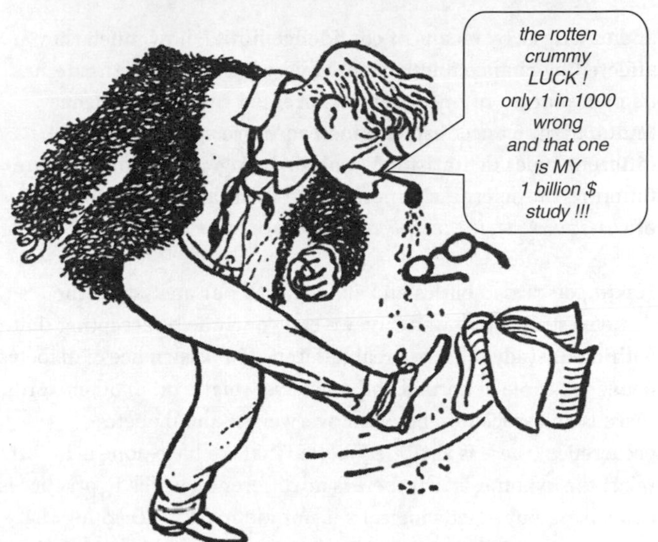

4. Calm down! No one can tell whether the wrong result is in yours or somebody else's study. And, please pay much more attention to sources of errors other than chance

Higher levels of confidence can be adopted, for example 99% or 99.9%, entailing only 1% or a 0.1% risk of being wrong, but the price paid for a higher degree of confidence is that the interval within which the difference can be stated to lie becomes larger.

Parameters and their estimates

For the general purpose of making inferences based on the data collected in an epidemiological study, incidence rates, risks, differences in rates or risks, means, and so on can be thought of as *parameters* characteristic of an ideal population, each parameter having a 'true' but unknown value. The empirical data make it possible to compute *estimates* of these parameters and to assess, by means of confidence limits, how much they are affected by chance fluctuations. Every parameter estimate has its own margin of uncertainty expressed by the confidence limits. Significance tests are instead more specific for the different types of statistical analysis being carried out and are found in the scientific papers in the form and under the names of *chi-square test*, *t test*, *F test*, and others.

Having discarded biases and chance with our analysis of the diabetes study in Flower City, we can conclude by accepting that within our study there is a real difference in occurrence of diabetes between people of normal and excessive weight, or, in other words, there is an association between overweight and diabetes occurrence (there is a subtlety here: what we have done is in fact reject the hypothesis that there is no difference, which in practice is equivalent, but strictly logically is not identical to accepting that there is a real difference). It remains to interpret the nature of this association: is it causal?; is overweight a determinant of diabetes?

Chapter 4
Establishing the causes of a disease

It may seem surprising that after a careful scrutiny to reasonably exclude biases and chance, the association established in a study between an exposure like overweight and a disease like diabetes should not automatically be taken to mean that overweight is a cause of diabetes. There are three reasons for this. First, the best that can be done in any observational study is to control for what is known, i.e. accurately measurable interfering factors (confounders) and known sources of selection or observation biases that can be ruled out or corrected. Nothing can be done to control for unknown factors that may have spuriously created the association, and for the free living subjects in the study – not rats in the tightly controlled conditions of a laboratory experiment – there is an endless list of such factors. Second, chance is ruled out based on the calculation of confidence limits or, much less preferably, significance tests that are in error once out of twenty or a hundred or a thousand occasions: there is never certainty. Third, more subtle but more fundamental, all types of analyses of the data from a study are explicitly or implicitly based on models. A simple, direct comparison of the incidence rates in two groups of people means that we implicitly believe in a model in which there are no confounding factors, not even age and gender, requiring adjustment. If instead we adjust for some confounding factors, we use a more complex model that involves a specific procedure with its assumptions, e.g. that the different factors operate by adding to or instead multiplying their contribution to the incidence rate. Different adjustments derive from using one or the other model. Similarly, we use models like tossing a perfectly balanced coin to calculate probabilities in order to arrive at confidence limits or significance tests, but events in real life may behave only roughly like balanced coins, introducing some unrecognizable error in our results. For these reasons, any association between an exposure and a disease that is reasonably well established in a study needs to go through a process of interpretation before a conclusion can be drawn about its nature, causal or non-causal.

A guide to interpreting associations

The problem of interpreting well-established associations came to a critical pass in the early 1960s, when a number of epidemiological studies had been accumulating that seriously indicted tobacco smoking as the culprit of several diseases, notably lung cancer. Up to that time, the so-called 'Koch's postulates' had been used as a common yardstick to evaluate associations between exposure and disease. Robert Koch, a key figure in the microbiological revolution of medicine, had discovered the bacteria causing tuberculosis and cholera, and formulated his criteria in 1890 to tackle the question: how can we distinguish, out of the thousands of micro-organisms hosted by any human body, the minority capable of producing disease from the great majority of innocuous parasites? In Koch's criteria, the decisive element permitting the interpretation of the association of a micro-organism with a human disease as causal was the laboratory reproduction of the disease in some experimental animal. When applied to the smoking/lung cancer issue, this criterion represented an insurmountable obstacle as no one had yet succeeded in inducing lung cancer by forcing animals to inhale tobacco smoke.

In 1962, a report of the Royal College of Physicians of the United Kingdom strongly endorsed the view that tobacco smoking causes lung cancer, but it was only with the 1964 report 'Smoking and Health' commissioned by the United States Surgeon General (head of the Public Health Service) to a panel of ten scientists that the issue of criteria for establishing causality was explicitly discussed. The report, produced after an in-depth examination of all the available evidence and the consultation of about 200 experts, stands as a masterpiece in the evaluation of scientific, and in particular epidemiological, evidence. The scientists enunciated and applied a number of principles to assess the meaning, causal or non-causal, of associations. At about the same time, Austin Bradford Hill from the London School of Hygiene and Tropical Medicine independently outlined similar principles in a profound and terse paper, stressing that they should be employed not as criteria to be invariably fulfilled, but rather as a guide in forming judgements of causality. These principles, either in their original forms or in one of the several subsequent variants, remain a suitable frame of reference to interpret exposure–disease associations.

In my own variant for this book, the guidelines consist of eight questions:

1 *Did the exposure precede the disease?* For example, was the past diet as reported by patients with colon cancer antecedent to the cancer, or were they in fact and inadvertently providing information on diets already modified because of minor symptoms of a silently developing cancer? Only diet prior to cancer onset can act as a cause or as a protective factor and, unless unequivocal information on this point is acquired, no conclusion about the nature of the diet–colon cancer association can be made.

2 *How strong is the association?* For the Flower City cohort in Chapter 3, we estimated the incidence rate of type 2 diabetes in overweight people as 18.5 per 1,000 person-years and in normal

weight people as 8.3, a difference of 10.2, with a 95% probability that the real difference would be between 2.0 and 18.3. As an alternative to this rate difference, we can compute a rate ratio of $18.5/8.3 = 2.2$, for which the 95% confidence limits turn out to be 1.2 and 5.4. The relative rate, or equivalently the ratio of risks (risk ratio, relative risk), is a much preferable tool for assessing the strength of an association than the risk difference, as errors from a variety of sources tend to be proportional to the rates and their possible role in producing an observed association is much better gauged by the ratio than by the difference. The same rate difference of $18.5 - 8.3 = 10.2$ per 1,000 person-years found in Flower City could hypothetically derive from two other rates, say 120.5 and 110.3. However, the first association implies a rate increase of $(10.2/8.2) \times 100 = 124\%$, while for the second, the increase is only $(10.2/110.3) \times 100 = 9\%$. The latter association may be accounted for easily by a 10% error, an amount not uncommon in epidemiological studies due to uncontrollable factors, while the former is much stronger as it greatly exceeds (by some 12 times) a 10% error. The best way of making the different strengths of the two associations immediately visible is to express them not through the rate difference (the same for both) but through the rate ratio (respectively 2.2 and 1.09). In general, the stronger a rate ratio or a risk ratio, the more confident one can be that it is unlikely to be due to errors. There is, however, no line, fixed for all studies, separating 'weak' and 'strong' rate ratios, as the amount of errors that can creep into different studies depends on their type, method of measurement employed, and population recruited.

3 *Does the association become stronger with increasing exposure?* It is reasonable to expect that if an exposure causes a disease, the incidence rate will rise with increasing levels of exposure. For example, the rate of lung cancer increases with the number of cigarettes smoked daily and with the number of years of smoking, two different aspects of the magnitude of the exposure.

4 *Is the association consistent?* Again, it is reasonable to expect that if an exposure causes a disease it will manifest this effect consistently,

if not in exactly the same way, in different subgroups of people, i.e. males and females, urban and rural dwellers, and so on.

5 *Is the association specific?* A strong association specific for a particular disease speaks in favour of a causal effect via a specific biological mechanism, whereas multiple weak associations with disparate diseases raise the suspicion that they may be an artefact due to some bias affecting the ensemble of a study.

6 *Is the association consistent with other biological evidence?* In the case of lung cancer, experiments to reproduce the disease by having animals inhale tobacco smoke failed for a long time. However, extracts of the smoke were repeatedly shown to cause cancer when painted on the skin of laboratory animals. This type of indirect evidence was rightly regarded as supporting the idea that tobacco smoking is capable of producing cancer. For the association between overweight and incidence of diabetes, there are biological mechanisms, particularly the fact that an excess of body fat interferes with the action of insulin, supporting the contention that overweight is a cause of diabetes.

7 *Has the association any analogue?* This may be the case, for example, when the exposure under study is the molecule of a chemical pollutant with a structure analogous to the molecule of an already known carcinogen.

8 *Is the association coherent across different studies?* An association that is repeatedly found in epidemiological studies of different types and in different populations is much more likely to be causal than an association showing up occasionally. This interpretation is further supported if cessation of exposure, as when smokers give up the habit, is followed by a decrease of the associated disease.

Schematically it can be stated that a positive answer to question number 1 is a must for an exposure–disease association to be judged causal; that a positive answer to question number 8 offers the strongest support to this judgement; and that a positive answer to each of questions 2 to 7 increases the likelihood that an association is causal.

If at this point you feel that the process of establishing an exposure–disease association and of judging its nature, causal or non-causal, is laborious and hardly simple, you are right; it is rigorous as well. You will also have realized how futile is the comment – frequently put forward to disqualify epidemiological investigations of environmental or other hazards – that epidemiological studies produce only 'soft' or 'statistical' evidence. What they produce is just scientific evidence, no more and no less than any other kind of correctly conducted scientific study.

Negative studies

Not finding an association when it was expected is the other side of the coin to finding an association between an exposure and a disease and going through the punctilious process of establishing whether it is causal. Particularly when the expectation was based on repeated results of previous epidemiological studies or on sound results from laboratory studies, a systematic scrutiny is needed of the reasons why no association turned up in a study. Several reasons fall under the heading of 'insufficient': insufficient number of subjects in the study, leading to what is called low 'power' to detect an increase in risk associated with the exposure; insufficient intensity or duration of exposure to induce an observable increase in risk, as may happen with pollutants recently introduced into the environment at low concentrations; insufficient period of observation, as effects like cancer usually appear many years after the onset of the exposure; finally, insufficient variation in exposure between the different groups of people to be compared, making it difficult to detect differences in risk between the groups. In addition, confounders and sources of bias, for example losses of records not occurring at random, can not only create spurious associations but also operate in the opposite direction by masking existing associations. The process of understanding why an expected association did not show up is no less lengthy, laborious, and complex than the process of establishing and judging the nature of an association.

In a nutshell, the basic principle is to distinguish clearly between 'no evidence of effect', that may often occur because no proper study has been done (whatever the reasons), and 'evidence of no effect' as emerging from adequate studies. The latter is reassuring while the former is simply uninformative. Thus studies in small communities, as often carried out to assuage legitimate concerns about risks from environmental factors, may be capable of excluding large excess risks but incapable of providing information about possible smaller excesses. A related principle is that the finding of a weak effect, for example a minor increase in asthma risk in people exposed to a chemical, cannot be taken as an

Necessary and sufficient causes

'The key point is that even if smoking were to be causally related to any disease it is neither a necessary nor a sufficient cause.' This statement, pronounced in a court by an expert 30 years after the publication of the 'Smoking and Health' report that established tobacco smoking as a cause of several diseases, is at the same time correct and misleading. Correct because, for instance, not all lung cancers occur in smokers (although the great majority do), nor do all smokers develop lung cancer. Misleading because it suggests that the only 'real' causes of diseases are those that are indispensable to produce all cases, or sufficient to trigger the disease every time they are present, or both. Causes that are necessary and sufficient, or just sufficient, are in fact uncommon in nature, being essentially represented by those inherited genes that constantly produce a genetic disease, such as the bleeding anomaly of haemophilia. Necessary causes are common in the field of infectious diseases, where only the presence of a specific micro-organism defines the disease (e.g. whatever the symptoms, there is no case of tuberculosis without the tuberculosis mycobacterium). Outside these domains, the great majority of causes of disease are, like tobacco smoking, neither necessary nor sufficient, yet they increase, often substantially, the probability (risk) of the disease, and removing or neutralizing them is highly beneficial. As an example, overweight and obesity, discussed before, are causes of diabetes but are neither necessary nor sufficient. In epidemiology, the general term *determinant* is used as synonymous of cause without prejudicing the detailed nature of the cause, whether necessary, sufficient, broad, like a type of diet or an occupation, or narrow, like a specific vitamin within the diet or a specific exposure to a chemical pollutant within an occupational setting.

indication that the chemical is in itself a weak, hence nearly innocuous, agent because the observable effect depends also on the study characteristics and on the dose of the chemical. Again 'evidence of a weak effect' cannot be taken automatically as 'evidence of a weak toxic agent'.

Individual and population determinants of disease

Recognizing that a factor like tobacco can cause lung cancer hinges on two conditions. First, and rather obviously, on tobacco being actually capable of producing the disease. Second, and less obviously, on how much smoking habits vary within the population being studied by the epidemiologist. If everybody smoked exactly 20 cigarettes per day from the ages of 15 to 45, there would be no difference in risk due to tobacco. Tobacco, although the dominant determinant of lung cancer in a population in which everybody smokes, would go completely unrecognized as a cause of the disease. Other factors, such as individual susceptibility, would be the only recognizable determinants by which people in a population with a high and uniform risk due to smoking stand out as being at an even higher risk. The conclusion would be reached that lung cancer is due to individual susceptibility, itself mostly dependent on the genes inherited from the parents: hence lung cancer would come to be regarded as an essentially genetic disease.

This fictional example was proposed in 1985 by Geoffrey Rose in an insightful article ('Sick individuals and sick populations') to clarify the distinction between individual and population determinants of disease. Population determinants, like the uniform smoking habit of the example, are responsible for the overall disease risk in a population, while individual determinants, like the individual susceptibilities, are responsible for the different risks between individuals or groups of individuals within the population. Studies comparing disease risk in groups within a population are suitable to identify the latter, but recognizing determinants that act essentially at the level of the whole population requires analysing and comparing risks between populations of different regions or countries or in the same populations at distinct times. No new principles need to be introduced to these analyses, but they may prove even more complex than those already outlined for studying associations and judging causality within a population.

Because of their general impact, population determinants are of major importance for health. A striking current case that follows the lines of the imaginary tobacco example is overweight and especially its highest degree, obesity. Excess weight basically originates from an imbalance between too many food calories ingested and too little expenditure of those calories through physical activity. Here excessive calorie consumption is the relevant exposure; if everybody or the great majority of the population is exposed nearly uniformly to some (not necessarily large) excess of calories from childhood, as tends to occur today in many high-income countries, the risk of obesity would be similarly high for everybody in the population. However, as in the smoking example, some people will be at an even higher risk than the average due to individual susceptibility, which becomes the main recognizable determinant of obesity. This is what is happening today as 'obesity genes' related to individual susceptibility are discovered, one after the other. They resonate in the media, and even in the scientific press, as the finally (for how long?) found and real causes of obesity. Focusing on genes is scientifically challenging, but it leads us astray if it ignores the main determinant of the overall population risk of obesity, i.e. widespread excessive intake of calories.

Other population determinants have an evident relevance. Polluted waters are a prime scourge in many low-resource countries, causing almost two million deaths worldwide every year. Air pollution affects the health of town dwellers in high- as in middle- and low-income countries. Less evidently, vaccination for a number of diseases such as measles or polio is essentially a population rather than an individual determinant of health and disease. Vaccination is certainly beneficial to the individual, but for most people the risk of the disease may already be low even without the vaccination. Vaccination, however, creates a 'herd immunity' or group immunity, whereby the chain of transmission of an infectious disease like measles is interrupted, bringing down to almost nil (or nil) the risk for the totality of the population. Other factors, such as being employed or unemployed, low or high level of education, have been known for quite some time to influence directly the health of individuals. More recent studies, however, show that the level of employment or of schooling in a society also acts indirectly as a population determinant of health. As we will see in Chapter 9, different types of interventions, targeted on single individuals or collectively on the material or social environment, are required to control individual and population determinants of disease.

Tobacco and health

Research on tobacco and health has been a key stimulus for the development of methods of modern epidemiology, including the principles for identifying causes of disease. The curves illustrating survival in smokers versus non-smokers (Figure 5) fix two moments in the unfolding of epidemiological research, nearly half a century apart.

There is a striking resemblance between the curves, summarizing how long smokers and non-smokers live, but they reflect fundamentally different statuses of knowledge. In 1938, not much was known epidemiologically and the US male curve solicited research to find out why the survival of smokers appeared to be so much poorer. The curves from the cohort of British doctors instead clearly show the result of all the diseases that in the meantime had been shown by epidemiological studies to be consequences of smoking.

The year 1950 marks a turning point in this research. Three important scientific papers were published in 1950: by Richard Doll and Austin Bradford Hill in the United Kingdom, by Ernest Wynder and Evarts Graham in the United States, and by Morton Levin, Hyman Goldstein, and Paul Gerhardt also in the United States. They are the first rigorous analytical studies of a disease, lung cancer, in relation to tobacco smoking. All three found a much higher frequency of smokers among lung cancer cases than among control subjects. These findings prompted a rapidly increasing number of epidemiological studies on the relation between smoking and cancers of the lung, other respiratory organs, and other diseases such as chronic bronchitis and myocardial infarction. Soon after their 1950 paper on lung cancer, Doll and Hill, in 1951, enrolled a cohort of some 40,000 British doctors to be followed for several decades recording mortality from different diseases. The choice of doctors had the advantage of involving a population that was rather homogeneous in socio-economic status and not exposed to other airborne toxic agents, unlike workers in many industries. The study stands as a cornerstone in epidemiology and similar follow-up studies on smoking were developed in other populations.

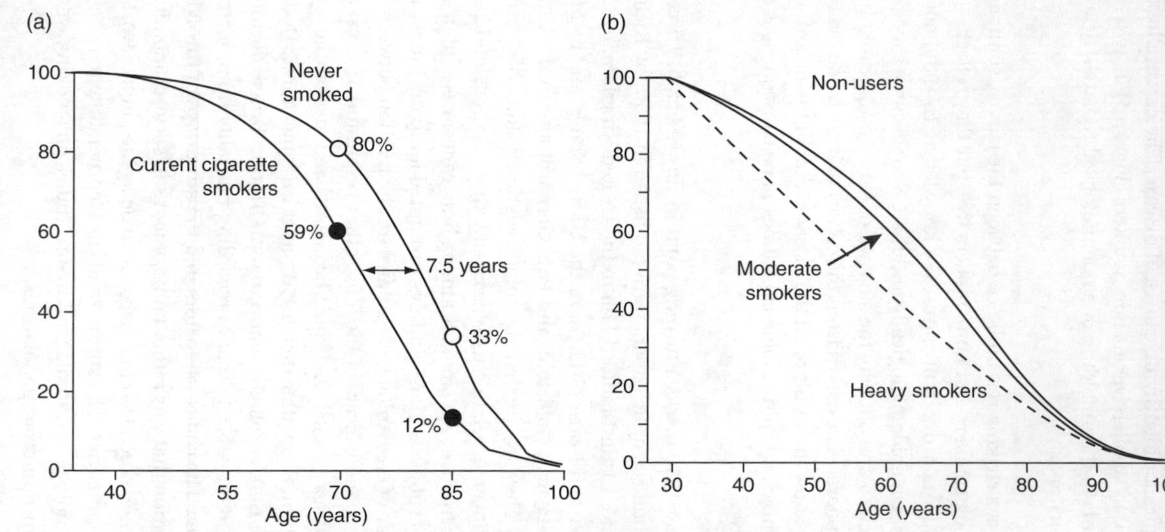

5. Percentage survival of British doctors 1951–1991 (left) and American men in the 1930s (right)

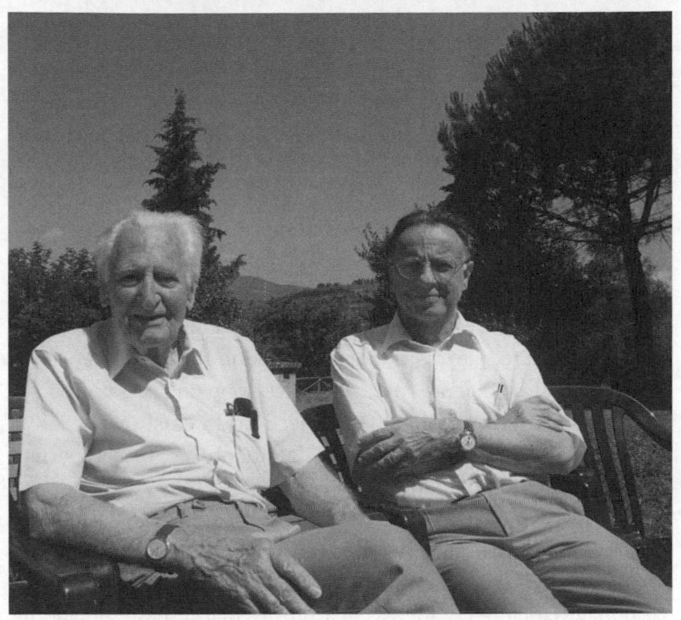

6. Sir Richard Doll (1912–2005) is the most eminent epidemiologist of the second half of the 20th century whose studies contributed fundamental knowledge on the causes of cancer. Here in 1998 with the book's author at the European Educational Programme in Epidemiology summer school in Florence where he lectured from 1993 to 2003

In addition, smoking became a factor to be measured in almost every epidemiological investigation because it could often be a confounder of the effects of other factors. As a result, a mass of information has been accumulating and continues to accumulate to the present day. A 2002 panel of the International Agency for Research on Cancer listed more than 70 main long-term follow-up studies that have investigated smoking-related diseases.

As the survival curve in (a) shows, the point in time at which half (i.e. 50% on the vertical axis) of all subjects alive at the age of 40 are still alive is reached 7.5 years earlier for current smokers than for lifetime non-smokers. In other words, smokers lose on average 7 years of life with respect to never smokers, and those who die between the ages of 35 and 69 lose an average of 22 years. In high-income countries, about one-fifth of all deaths are caused by tobacco smoking, which is responsible worldwide for more than five million deaths every year – more than half of them in middle- and low-income countries. By far the largest proportion of the 1.3 billion smokers in the world today is in these countries, and because the full-blown effects of smoking become manifest after two to three decades of continuing smoking, a huge increase in tobacco-related deaths is to be expected in the future in middle- and low-income countries unless smoking cessation is successfully implemented. Some projections forecast that in 2020 there will be 9 million deaths due to tobacco, three-quarters of them in middle- and low-income countries.

A range of diseases contributes to this toll: cancers of at least 13 organs (including lung, nasal passages, larynx, pharynx, mouth, oesophagus, bladder, pancreas), cardiovascular diseases, including heart attacks and stroke, and chronic obstructive pulmonary disease ('chronic bronchitis'). These results are not surprising because tobacco smoke contains almost 5,000 identified chemicals, many of them toxic and more than 50 definitely carcinogenic. Many of these substances are also found in the second-hand smoke that goes into the environment around smokers to which other people, including non-smokers, are passively exposed. Passive smoking is associated with an increase in risk of several diseases in non-smokers ranging from respiratory ailments in children to myocardial infarction. For lung cancer, more than 50 studies support a causal role of passive smoking involving an increase in risk of about 25%.

Tobacco smoking has emerged as the greatest killer in peacetime. All forms of tobacco use, including pipe smoking, chewing, and sniffing, are noxious even if with less pervasive and strong effects than cigarette smoking. This gloomy picture is brightened by the fact that preventive efforts, involving a combination of measures, educational campaigns, increasing taxation on tobacco products, and prohibition of smoking in public places, have translated into reduction of tobacco use in several high-income countries. Young people have been less prone to take up smoking habits and appreciable numbers of people have stopped smoking. Duration of exposure to tobacco smoke is crucial for risk, hence the later one starts to smoke (short of not starting at all) and the sooner one manages to stop, the better the health prospect. Stopping at any age is beneficial: in people who started to smoke in early youth, stopping at age 30 reduces the risk of developing lung cancer before age 75 to nearly that of non-smokers, and even stopping at age 50 reduces the risk to one-third with respect to continuing smokers.

Chapter 5
Testing how to control a disease

Observational and experimental studies

The principles of epidemiology hitherto outlined apply to all studies, although the examples and the discussion have focused on observational studies, in which the investigator intervenes only by observing people and recording information at a point in time or during a time period. The great advantage of this type of study is that it can in principle be carried out in all contexts to investigate any health phenomenon. The disadvantage is that all comparisons between rates and risks in different groups of people, for example rates of chronic bronchitis among those exposed to air pollutants in a city and those not exposed, can always be influenced by unknown factors other than the pollutants. The elaborate procedures outlined in the previous chapters are necessary in these observational situations to reach conclusions about the possible causal role of an exposure such as air pollution on a disease such as chronic bronchitis.

Life would be simpler if the epidemiologist could choose, as in a laboratory experiment, which subjects would be assigned polluted and unpolluted air to breathe for several years, making sure in advance that all subjects in the experiment were closely similar in all respects, except for the 'treatment', i.e. exposure to different types of air. The simplest and safest device to achieve this similarity would consist in assigning the subjects perfectly at random, by tossing a coin, to breathing polluted or unpolluted air. The random assignment would act as an insurance against all known and, crucially important, unknown factors that could make the two groups of people different. Clearly this randomized experiment, or *randomized controlled trial (RCT)*, is not feasible, both for ethical and technical reasons. Hence the lesser scope of experimental randomized studies (also generically and less accurately called 'intervention studies') in respect to observational studies, notably when an agent, like polluted air, is investigated because of possible adverse effects on health. The elective place of the randomized experiment is in investigating agents which may have beneficial health effects. Promising new drugs are continuously tested on population of patients affected by a great range of diseases, from all kinds of cancer to heart diseases like myocardial infarction and angina pectoris to rheumatic diseases. In addition to these trials of treatment, large randomized experiments are carried out in healthy populations to test preventive interventions. Screening programmes for early diagnosis and treatment of serious conditions such as breast or colon cancer are tested in population randomized experiments and new vaccines – for example, against AIDS – are commonly tested using randomized trials in large populations.

The first vaccine against poliomyelitis

Until the middle of the last century, poliomyelitis, or infantile paralysis, was an infectious disease of the nervous system occurring especially in summer in epidemic waves, irregular in intensity. It affected particularly children and young people, who might experience only a transient fever or instead suffer lifelong flaccid paralysis of the limbs, or die if the nervous centres controlling respiration were attacked by the virus causing the disease. Three types of the virus had been identified. Some small-scale but unsuccessful attempts with vaccines had been made when, in the early 1950s, a very promising vaccine to be administered by intra-muscular injection was developed by Dr Jonas Salk at the University of Pittsburgh. It consisted of a 'killed' virus that had lost its ability to produce the disease while retaining the power to stimulate a protective immunity in the body of the vaccinated subjects.

Before recommending the vaccine for mass administration, sound evidence of its actual efficacy was needed. Just starting to administer the vaccine and seeing whether the incidence rate was declining was not an option as the disease frequency varied too much from one year to the next. It would have been impossible to distinguish a decrease due to the vaccine from spontaneous variation. An additional problem was the difficulty in correctly diagnosing as poliomyelitis, rather than for example 'flu', the numerous minor cases which were the main source of the spread by direct contact between people. The decision was then taken to implement a true prevention experiment on primary school children.

Children aged 6 to 9, whose parents had agreed to take part in the study, had to be assigned at random to receive the vaccine or a no-vaccine treatment. They were recruited in 84 counties of 11 states across the whole territory of United States. The number of participants had to be very large, so that even if the vaccine gave only a 50% protection, a difference in the incidence rate between the vaccinated and the unvaccinated group would be detectable with a high degree of confidence. One dose of the vaccine against all three types of the virus had to be administered at the start of the study, a second dose one week later, and a third after five weeks. The no-vaccine treatment consisted of three injections but of an inactive preparation strictly similar in appearance to the vaccine, i.e. a *placebo*. When feasible, placebo treatments are the best form of comparison for an active medication as it is well established that simply receiving an inactive medication may produce an effect. One may wonder, however, whether ethics committees would today approve injecting children three times with an inactive preparation. The trial was 'double blinded' as not only the children (and their families) did not know whether they were receiving the vaccine or the inactive preparation, but their physicians were also unaware of which treatment was administered. In this way, they would not be influenced at all by knowledge of the treatment when, confronted with a suspect case, they would have to decide about a diagnosis of poliomyelitis. Close to 400,000 children whose parents had given consent were entered into the trial (200,745 vaccinated and 201,229 unvaccinated) out of a total of about 750,000 in the areas where the trial took place. 82 cases of poliomyelitis were observed among the vaccinated children in the six months after vaccination, i.e. a risk of 41 per 100,000 and almost double, 162 cases, were observed among the unvaccinated, a risk of 81 per 100,000. The difference between the two risks, $81-41 = 40$ is larger than would be expected by chance if there was no real difference. An even stronger decrease was noted for the more serious form (paralytic) of the disease, with risks of 16 per 100,000 in the vaccinated group and 57 per 100,000 in the non-vaccinated. The conclusion here is much more straightforward than in the case of an observational study. Because the children were assigned at random to vaccination and no-vaccination, the two groups should be closely similar in all respects except for the difference in treatment, which can be confidently regarded as the cause of the decreased rate among the vaccinated children. The trial demonstrated the effectiveness of the vaccine and initiated programmes of systematic vaccination all over the world. The Salk vaccine is even today considered to be the most effective and safe protection against poliomyelitis.

Five key features of randomized controlled trials

1 The *study design* is always based on randomization, usually implemented today by means of computer-generated lists of random numbers. People can just be assigned at random to the different treatments or some additional condition can be introduced. For instance, in a trial of nicotine patches for smoking cessation, subjects were randomly assigned to different types of patches or to a placebo within each centre participating in the study. In this way, correct comparisons of treatments became possible not only overall on the pooled data from all centres but also within each of the centres located in different countries.

2 The choice of *the study population* is critical for generalizing the conclusions drawn from a trial. In the nicotine patches experiment, volunteer subjects were recruited who had made two or more previous unsuccessful attempts and who were going to receive advice by a physician. The conclusion of the trial, that the patches effectively increase the probability of stopping smoking, would not necessary apply to less motivated people. Moreover, treatments that have been shown to be effective and safe in adults may not work in the same way in old people or children. As a general principle, a treatment (e.g. a drug) for a specific disease should be prescribed only in subjects closely similar to those in the trials that have demonstrated its efficacy. The incessant pressure from the pharmaceutical industry to extend the use of a drug to other diseases should be resisted until there is clear evidence that it works for them as well. To be informative, a trial should include a sufficient number of subjects. What a 'sufficient' number is can be calculated at the planning stage based on the size of the difference between treatments one wishes to detect with a high degree of confidence. If one is interested in picking up only a very large effect, for example the complete elimination of a disease by a vaccine, a relatively small number will be adequate because if such a major effect exists, it is likely to show up in any event. If at the opposite end one wishes to show that a new vaccine that is cheaper and easier to administer is

not (or only minimally) different in efficacy from the best vaccine hitherto available, a very large number of subjects will be required to exclude the possibility that the new vaccine is not inferior, even by a small but still statistically significant amount, to the old one.

3 The *treatment* can be as simple as a drug or a vaccine or much more complex, such as an intervention to modify the habitual diet. A recent randomized trial in this field showed that a reduction in the intake of calories could reduce weight in volunteer subjects keeping their amount of physical activity nearly constant. Remarkably, it also showed that the composition of the diet did not matter, whether high or low (within reasonable limits) in fat, protein, or sugars, provided the diet was low in caloric content. Keeping to the diet within the trial implied, however, repeated contact and strict surveillance of the subjects, something that may not be easily reproduced in the population. Basically, a randomized trial is justified when there is genuine uncertainty about the effect of a treatment in respect to a placebo or to another already established treatment. This uncertainty materializes a condition of 'equipoise' between the treatments.

4 Usually several *responses* to the treatment or *endpoints* will be assessed to measure the intended and the possible adverse effects of the treatment. The incidence rate of myocardial infarction may be measured in a trial testing a drug aimed at its prevention but any other anomalous manifestation will also be carefully monitored as it may indicate an adverse effect of the drug. The best device to avoid all conscious and unconscious influences on the observation and recording of the endpoints is to keep both subjects and physicians blind to the treatments administered. This may not always be possible as, for example, when the treatments are diets of different compositions.

5 The *analysis of the data* collected during the study is done at the planned end of it. Often, however, some intermediate analyses can be done to monitor what is happening: if early indications of an obvious advantage of one of the treatments

emerge, it may become unethical to continue with the other and inferior treatments; or if signs of serious adverse effects show up, it may become necessary to stop the trial. Because of these delicate implications, the intermediate analyses are usually placed in the hands of a trial-monitoring committee independent of the investigators responsible for the study. A particular type of analysis is not infrequently necessary to take into account the fact that a proportion of trial participants will abandon their assigned treatment during the course of the trial. Most likely these drop-outs do not occur by chance but because, for instance, some subjects find it too cumbersome to adhere to a diet, or simply dislike it. In these circumstances, a comparison of the effects of different diets on, for example, the incidence rates of diabetes between people who kept to their diet throughout the trial would not reflect the reality. A more realistic analysis, named *by intention to treat*, will compare the diabetes rates between the groups of people as initially assigned to each diet, regardless of whether some people dropped out in each group. In fact, the net effect of a diet as it may be proposed, if beneficial, to the whole population will be the result from the combination of the effects among those who adhere to it and whatever other effect ensues among those who started it but then switched to other regimes.

Randomized, non-randomized, and spontaneous experiments

Randomized trials are a precious tool in medical and epidemiological research. They can be looked at from two slightly different angles. From one viewpoint, they are the instrument to test how effective a treatment is. Before the era of the randomized control trial, heralded by the British trial of streptomycin on pulmonary tuberculosis in 1948, the evidence of the positive and negative effects of a treatment was essentially based on the accumulation of clinical experience supported by knowledge from physiology and pathology.

In epidemiology the evidence of how, for instance, a vaccine worked was based on observational studies. Compared to randomized trials, these methods are more cumbersome, as they require a large accumulation of concordant results from clinical or epidemiological observations before any sound conclusions can be drawn, and less sensitive, because minor but medically important effects – say, a 5–10% reduction in the incidence rate of a disease – cannot be recognized with any confidence. The randomized trial has therefore become the generally accepted standard for testing treatments, preventive or remedial.

From another angle, the randomized trial is the acid test of causality. Removal of a presumed cause of a disease conducted in the form of a randomized trial is the best proof that the exposure is indeed a cause. This test may sometimes be feasible. For example, a vaccination programme against the hepatitis B virus could not be introduced all at once in the whole population of newborns in the Gambia. This unfavourable circumstance was turned into an actual advantage by picking the children to be vaccinated first at random, so allowing a correct comparison with the unvaccinated children born in the same year (by the fourth year, the vaccination reached all newborns in the country). The expected reduction in liver cancer among the vaccinated children once they become adult should provide conclusive evidence that the hepatitis B virus causes not only hepatitis – an established fact – but liver cancer, the most frequent cancer in many countries of Africa and South East Asia.

For many exposures clearly indicated to be harmful by observational studies and laboratory experiments, a planned randomized removal of the exposure is neither feasible nor ethical. A surveillance programme should nonetheless be set up to observe the course of disease following the 'natural experiment' of removing (in whatever way) the exposure. For instance, a substantial number of the doctors in the prospective study of Richard Doll and Austin Bradford Hill cited in Chapter 4 stopped smoking. Already within the first five years after stopping, the incidence rate of lung cancer fell by almost one-third, providing additional and strong evidence supporting the causal role of tobacco smoking.

When overall survival is examined, the experience of British doctors showed (Figure 7) that the sooner smoking is stopped the more an (ex)smoker can expect to live as long as a lifelong non-smoker. In plain terms, the best option is to never start smoking, the next best is to stop soon, and even stopping late produces at least some rapid benefit.

Well-designed, conducted, and analysed observational and randomized studies are two complementary instruments of epidemiology that contribute to advancing knowledge even when they produce contrasting results, as the case of vegetables and cancer shows. Thirty years ago, several observational studies had already indicated that the consumption of vegetables, a source of vitamin A, and blood levels of vitamin A higher than average were associated with a reduced risk of cancer. There was some evidence from laboratory experiments showing that vitamin A and its derived compounds in the body could inhibit the transformation and proliferation of normal cells into cancer cells. To test directly the causal hypothesis that vitamin A inhibits cancer, a randomized controlled trial was carried out on more than 8,000 adult smokers (particularly at risk of lung cancer) in Finland comparing a placebo treatment with the administration of beta-carotene, the precursor substance of vitamin A present in yellow vegetables and fruits. The results turned out to be opposite to the hopes. The trial had to be stopped because a surge of lung cancer showed up in the men receiving the beta-carotene. This could mean that beta-carotene given at the doses of the trial, appreciably higher than in a normal diet, had an adverse rather than a beneficial effect. It might also mean that in the previous observational studies, vitamin A was not responsible for the reduced risk of cancer but simply an indicator of other substances present in vegetables and capable of inhibiting cancer development. Even today, the protective

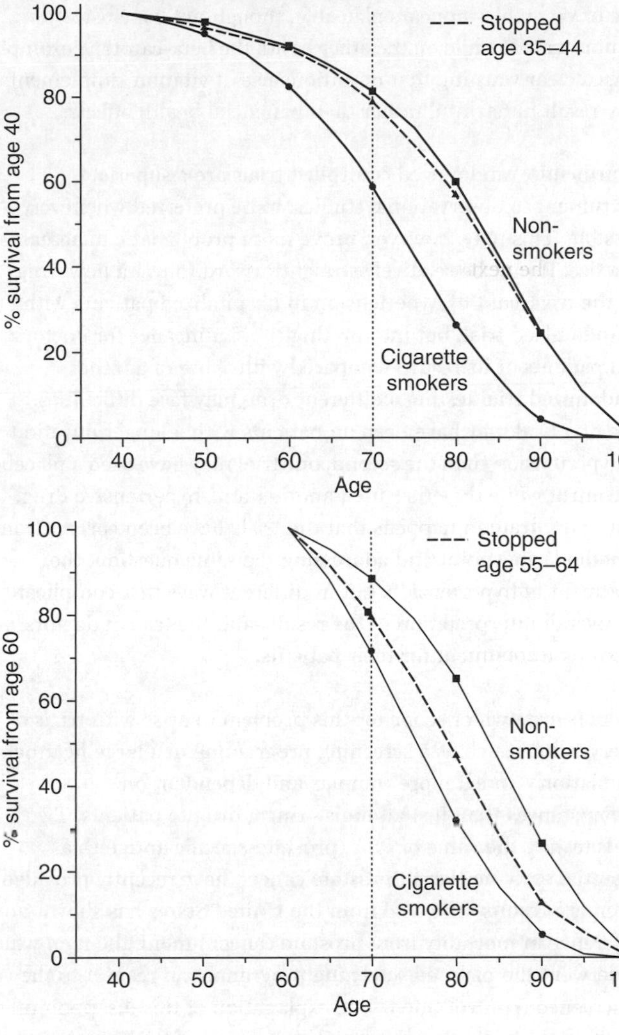

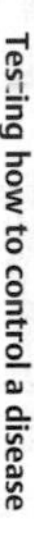

7. Stopping smoking at any age prolongs your life

role of vegetables appears plausible, though not conclusively demonstrated, while on the other hand, the beta-carotene example gives a clear warning that incautious use of vitamin supplements may result in harmful rather than beneficial health effects.

In principle, randomized controlled trials are a superior instrument to observational studies, to be preferred whenever possible. This may, however, prove more problematic in actual practice. It may be relatively straightforward to test a new drug for the treatment of hypertension in hospitalized patients with a randomized trial, but interpreting the significance for doctors and patients of its results compared with those of another randomized trial testing a different drug may face difficulties. The first trial may have been on patients with a longer duration of hypertension than the second, one trial may have used a placebo as control while the other used another anti-hypertensive drug, and so on. It often happens that the trials have been correct from a methods viewpoint and addressing the same question, the treatment of hypertension, but in different ways that complicate the overall interpretation of the results and the task of doctors choosing a treatment for their patients.

There is even wider scope for this problem to arise with trials of interventions such as a screening programme in a large healthy population – much more complex and dependent on circumstances than just administering a drug to patients. Two trials testing the value of PSA (prostate-specific antigen), a potential early marker of prostate cancer, have recently provided diverging results. The trial from the United States has shown no difference in mortality from prostate cancer among the men who underwent the planned screening programme in respect to the unscreened (control) men. One explanation of this disappointing result might be that a substantial proportion of the control group had spontaneously undergone an occasional PSA test, hence any difference between the screened and the control group might have been reduced to the point of becoming undetectable.

The trial from Europe in fact showed a reduction in mortality of about 20%. This, however, has to be weighed against the fact that of the 16% of men in which the PSA test was positive, 3 out of 4 were found to have no cancer after undergoing a prostate biopsy, a procedure neither too pleasant nor totally exempt from complications such as infection or bleeding. The question of the possible beneficial effect of PSA screening for prostate cancer remains completely open.

In the context of drug or vaccine testing, the randomized controlled trial is a 'Phase 3' experimental study comparing the drug or vaccine to a reference treatment (placebo or other drug). 'Phase 1' and 'Phase 2' precede the randomized trial. In 'Phase 1' experiments, the safety of the drug is usually explored by administering small but increasing doses to a limited number of volunteer subjects; data on absorption, distribution in the body, and elimination of the drug are also collected. Once a safe range of doses has been identified, 'Phase 2' experiments provide initial information on whether the drug has some of the intended beneficial effects. Again, a limited number of subjects is studied using rapidly obtained responses: for example, in the cancer field the reduction of the mass of a tumour will signal some efficacy of the drug, although the most relevant effect, to be explored in 'Phase 3' randomized trials, will be the patients' length of survival. These trials allow an evaluation of the *efficacy* of a treatment under ideal experimental conditions. When, however, the same treatment is applied in everyday practice, its actual effect, or *effectiveness*, will not only depend from its efficacy but also on how accurately the patients for whom it is indicated are identified, on how well they comply with the treatment, on whether they spontaneously recur to other treatments and on a variety of other life circumstances.

Chapter 6
Following up people's health

Observing people without intervening with treatments

In randomized controlled trials, subjects treated differently are followed up over time to observe the effects of the intervention (treatment). People can, however, be observed over time even when no treatment was administered at the start of the study period. We first encountered this type of study in Chapter 3 when comparing rates of onset of diabetes in overweight and normal-weight people. These purely observational follow-up studies are called *cohort studies*. A group of subjects is chosen, a number of characteristics (exposures) of the subject are measured and recorded, e.g. weight, blood pressure, diet, smoking habits. The subjects are then followed up in time, and a number of events recorded, typically the occurrence of a disease, like diabetes or myocardial infarction, or death from a disease or change in some trait like weight or blood pressure. A classical cohort study is the investigation of the health effects of tobacco in British doctors, which we met in Chapter 4, and again in Chapter 5. Cohort studies addressing possible short-term effects of exposures such as food poisoning may span days or weeks, while cohort studies investigating long-term effects, such as cancer or atherosclerosis, must necessarily last for decades, involving cumbersome logistics. As they unfold prospectively in the future, these studies are also known as *prospective cohort studies* or simply *prospective studies*. When all or some of the measurements made at the beginning are repeated over time, the study is often qualified as *longitudinal*. In recent years, a number of large cohort studies have been started to investigate three types of open questions about common diseases: the long-term positive and negative effects of diet; the role played by genetic factors; the influence of early life experiences, in the maternal womb and during childhood, on adult diseases.

A prototype contemporary study: the EPIC international investigation

The EPIC (European Prospective Investigation into Cancer) is a project currently jointly coordinated by the International Agency for Research on Cancer in Lyon, France (a research centre of the World Health Organization) and the Department of Public Health of the Imperial College in London. It initially focused on cancers in relation to nutrition but was soon expanded to other chronic diseases, like diabetes and myocardial infarction, and to genetics and environmental factors. It started with several preliminary studies developing and testing questionnaires on habitual diet and moved to recruiting adults, mostly in the age range 35 to 70, in 23 centres in 10 West European countries (Denmark, France, Germany, Greece, Italy, the Netherlands, Norway, Spain, Sweden, United Kingdom). Some 520,000 people entered the study between 1992 and 2000. Each provided detailed information on diet – collected using comparable procedures in the different countries – and other personal characteristics such as sex, age, education, alcohol and tobacco consumption, physical activity, reproductive history for women, previous diseases. Height, weight, and waist and hip circumferences (as indicators of fat distribution) were measured. Blood was taken from about 385,000 subjects for storage at -196°C in freezers filled with liquid nitrogen.

At this temperature, all biochemical reactions taking place in blood are blocked and the specimens can be stored without

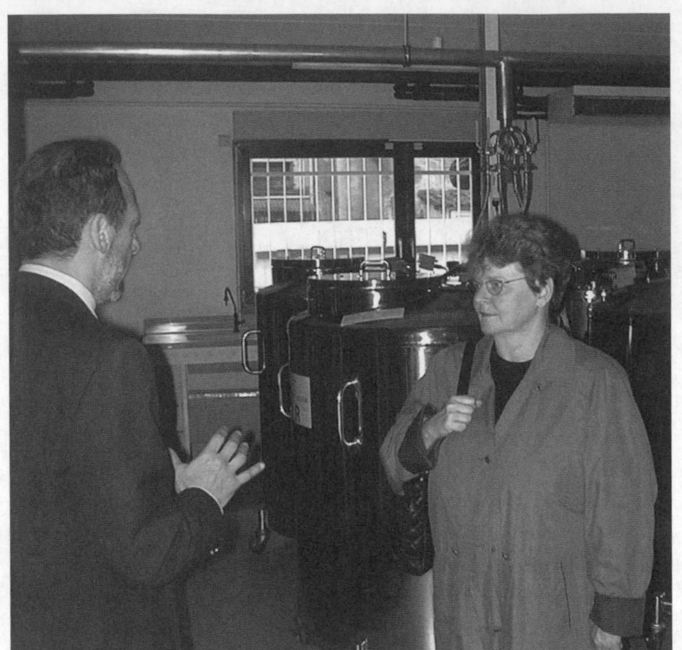

8. Dr Go Brundlant, Director General of the World Health Organization, visits the International Agency for Research on Cancer in Lyon. Dr Elio Riboli – currently chairman of Public Health at the Imperial College, London – describes the organization of the EPIC depository of biological specimens

alteration for years. The subjects are followed up, recording causes of death and the occurrence of cancers through permanent systems of cancer registration (Cancer Registries) where these exist or, for cancer as well as for other diseases, using physician or hospital records.

A wide range of specific studies is being conducted within the EPIC cohort and findings of major interest have already emerged. Nearly 15,000 deaths from any cause have been recorded and it has been shown that the distribution of fat in the body, in particular an increased deposit of fat in the abdomen translating into a large abdominal girth, predicts the risk of death. Another study found that the risk of cancer of the intestine (colon and rectum) is associated with high consumption of red and processed meat. In a third study, the risk of breast cancer occurring after menopause was shown to be related to the level of both female and male hormones in the blood, a caution against the use of male hormones (like testosterone) that had been proposed for prevention of bone fragility in post-menopausal women.

Each of the blood specimens stored in the EPIC depository contains different fractions: serum and plasma, in which many biochemical compounds can be analysed; envelopes of red cells, in which some substances like fatty acid molecules can be assayed; and most important, white blood cells that provide DNA for genetic studies. Genes are embodied as sequences of variable length of elementary molecules (nucleotides or bases, coupled as base-pairs) in the long molecules of DNA. These are in turn packed within the chromosomes included in a cell nucleus. Every human being receives 23 chromosomes from the father and 23 from the mother, each of these two sets containing more than three billion base-pairs. About 99% of these are common to all humans, but this leaves more than ten million nucleotides that can vary from one person to another. In these variations are hidden the differences in individual susceptibility to disease, a universe that has become accessible to direct exploration only recently, since the revolution in molecular biology and technology has made it possible first to measure and then to test the differences in the structure of individual nucleotides on a very large scale. Today, it is feasible to test a million nucleotides at once for variations in structure (form), in studies of 'single nucleotide polymorphisms' (SNPs) that cover all chromosomes, i.e. the whole 'genome'.

Within EPIC and in a fast-expanding number of other studies, associations are now sought between these genetic variations and disease, in the same way as in the past associations of smoking with disease were investigated. Testing hundreds of thousands or millions of associations, and understanding whether and in what way a gene variant causes a disease, involves three major challenges. First, it requires a very large number of cases of a disease, even beyond the numbers achievable in a project like EPIC: hence data from similar, albeit smaller, studies are combined with those of EPIC for 'consortium' analyses. Second, testing a million associations increases the number of them that turn out to be statistically significant at the commonly adopted levels of 5% or 1% probability of error. A 5% level implies that 50,000 associations will appear as statistically significant merely by chance! New methods of statistical analysis are being developed to keep this flurry of chance results under control. Third, and most complex, a single nucleotide variant will very rarely be found responsible 'per se' for individual susceptibility to developing a common disease like colon cancer or myocardial infarction. The action of multiple genes is likely and to unravel the puzzle of their cooperation combined with the influences of external factors like diet will require the investigation of the chains of events leading from the gene variants to gene expression into proteins, cellular functions, and finally to disease. For this task, resources like EPIC that make possible not only the testing of genetic polymorphisms in DNA but also the assaying of biochemical components such as proteins in serum and plasma, represent a precious research instrument.

Among studies broadly similar to EPIC, the British Biobank, which has started recruitment of subjects aged 40–69 in 2007, targets on a total of half a million. In Denmark, a 'Danish National Birth Cohort' recruited nearly 100,000 pregnant women between 1997 and 2002 with the main objective of investigating how the period from conception to early childhood influences the health conditions of adult life. Both projects have a collection of blood specimens, as do several other studies at the advanced frontier of today's epidemiology, combining the study of genetic and external factors – dietary, occupational, environmental, and social. As these ongoing projects show, the timescale of epidemiology is often long and very different from the time of weeks, months, or a few years taken by studies carried out in the laboratory using materials like cell cultures or experimental animals: the simple reason is that for finding out what happens and why it happens to people over a lifetime there is no real alternative to observing people over a lifetime.

The five key features of cohort studies

1 The choice of the *population* is crucial. Essentially the exposures that are the focus of investigation must be present and variable in intensity in the population, otherwise the study will be a waste of time and resources. There is little point in choosing a population where everybody eats similar diets for a study of diet and disease: for this reason, the EPIC investigation included a spectrum of countries from northern to southern Europe, where diets (still) exhibit sizeable differences. For the same reason, when investigating the possible health effects of an air pollutant like benzo-pyrene from heating, industrial, or vehicle exhausts, the first choice would be a population of, say, gas workers, some of whom were occupationally exposed at high levels in coal-firing, rather than a general urban population exposed to low and relatively uniform levels. A population may also be chosen because it shows a high frequency of a disease, for example liver cancer, or of a disease and an exposure, say liver cancer and hepatitis B. In this case, the purpose of the study is to find out whether the risk of liver cancer is indeed concentrated among people who had hepatitis. Cohorts of patients, for example those with chronic bronchitis, are special populations to be followed up in time after the first manifestations of the condition in order to understand the natural history of the disease development. This knowledge is indispensable to clinicians for formulating correct prognoses for individual patients.

2 The *study design* may include a cohort recruited in a single place, like the classic study in the small town of Framingham in

Massachusetts that has provided fundamental information on the determinants of cardiovascular diseases, or several cohorts, as in the EPIC project. The number of subjects to be recruited should in any case be sufficient to detect with high probability the risk of disease associated with different levels of an exposure, e.g. of myocardial infarction with amount of fat in the diet. For this reason, studies of workplace hazards often combine populations of workers at several plants, each of which employs too few workers exposed to a particular hazard to permit a meaningful investigation. Usually the age range and the gender of the people to be included in the cohort are also specified. Should the people actually in the cohort be a random sample representative of the chosen population? Because comparisons are made between groups within the cohort, for instance between people eating different amounts of fat, this is not an absolute requirement (although if the proportion of people invited who refuse to enter the study is high, various types of biases may creep in).

3 The *factors* or *exposures* to be measured belong to two categories. First, those that can be measured at the moment of people's entry into the study: education, profession, blood pressure, blood glucose level, present smoking habits, and so on. Second, those that reflect past experience, recent or remote: lifetime smoking habits, past jobs, diet during the last week or month or year, and so on. A proper standardization of the methods of measurement can ensure the quality of measurements for the first category, but it cannot completely prevent errors of recollection for the second category.

4 Events such as disease occurrence or death are the typical *responses* to be recorded in most cohort studies. Mechanisms for tracing the people in the cohort are essential: a cohort study in which the percentage of subjects of whom it is unknown whether they are still alive or dead is higher than 5% or, at worst, 10% is usually regarded as of mediocre quality. Existing national or local systems of death registration and disease (e.g. cancer) registries are used both for ascertaining the status of a person and the disease

diagnoses. When these systems are not in operation or are unreliable an active follow-up mechanism has to be put in place, for example through a network of the subjects' doctors.

5 The *analysis* of a cohort study is straightforward. Incidence rates or risks of disease are computed for groups with different exposures and the relative rates or relative risks encountered in Chapter 4 calculated to find out whether exposure–disease associations emerge. As many factors are at work, it will always be indispensable to adjust for several of them regarded as mere disturbances: for instance, when comparing the risk of lung cancer in people heavily and only slightly exposed to urban air pollution, it will be necessary to remove the influence of at least gender, age, and smoking habits. This can be done by the methods of logistic or Cox's and Poisson regression mentioned in Chapter 3. These methods, easy to employ today thanks to user-friendly statistical computer packages, should not be applied blindly, lest one removes effects that should be left in. For example, in a study of the role of dietary salt in the causation of stroke it would be appropriate to remove the influence of other factors such as gender, age, tobacco smoking, blood cholesterol, diabetes. On the other hand, it would be unwise to remove the influence of blood pressure because the direct effect of salt is to increase blood pressure which in turn influences stroke. To decide which factors need to be adjusted for is specific to each study and requires careful consideration of the possible relationships between factors.

The historical cohort study

Cohort studies are usually long-term investments (and people in the cohort may survive longer than the epidemiologists who initiate the study). A very advantageous short-cut, which has been used often in studying exposures in the workplace, is the 'historical cohort study'. When records of employment are available, a cohort can be formed of all workers entering employment say between 1930 and 1950, who are then followed up to the present, establishing whether they are alive or dead through national or local registries, and in the latter case the date and cause of the death. This design allows calculation of rates and risks like any prospective cohort study, the only difference being that the cohort is followed up in the past rather than in the future.

An early example of a well-conducted historical cohort study is the 1913 German investigation of nearly 20,000 children born to tubercular parents and more than 7,000 children born to non-tubercular parents which showed that children of tubercular parents had shorter lives than children of non-tubercular parents and that their increased mortality was in addition related to the number of siblings and to lower social class.

A classic example is the 1968 study of asbestos insulation workers in the two states of New York and New Jersey present at the end of 1943 or subsequently enrolled until the end of 1962 and followed up until the end of April 1967. Their mortality from any cause was double that of men of the same age in the general population. For lung cancer, the mortality of the workers was eight times higher and in addition more than one-tenth of the deaths were due to mesothelioma, a malignant tumour of the linings of lung (pleura) or intestine (peritoneum) that is extremely rare in the general population. These findings clearly demonstrate the danger of asbestos, all the more so as the results for lung cancer were adjusted to remove the influence of the workers' smoking habits. The study went even one step further: it showed that in workers jointly exposed to asbestos and tobacco smoking, the risk of lung cancer was much increased by a reciprocal strengthening of their separate effects. The increase in risk for lung cancer was, as mentioned, about eightfold, and the increase in risk from smoking about twelvefold: the increase in risk arising from the combined exposure turned out to be close to $8 \times 12 = 96$-fold. It was the first epidemiological evidence of how different factors can not only present as confounders of each other's effect within a study but can cooperate or 'interact' to produce strong joint effects.

Chapter 7
Investigating people's past experiences

The same information for much less work and cost

Large long-term cohort studies, like the international EPIC or the birth cohorts, need massive amounts of information on diet, smoking habits, occupation, and many other factors collected on each member of the cohorts to be processed in statistical analyses, a task that does not pose insurmountable problems today thanks to the availability of software and computing facilities. Much less tractable are the problems arising from the need to carry out multiple laboratory analyses on the stored blood specimens of hundreds of thousands of people. These can, however, be overcome by using only the blood specimens from a fraction or representative 'sample' of the cohort rather than from all its members (the same device is widely used for opinion polls). A sample that includes a number of subjects (not too small) can provide the same information as the whole cohort at a much reduced workload and expenditure. For example, to investigate how the blood levels of sex hormones in 1997 influence the subsequent risk of breast cancer, advantage can be taken within the EPIC cohort of the breast cancer cases accumulated during the follow-up until 2008. All these cases, or a randomly selected subgroup, are included in the sample and for each of them one or more control women are extracted from the cohort at random.

Usually a more elaborate sampling plan is adopted, for example by picking at random a control belonging to the same country, centre, and age group as a case. With four controls per case, this 'case-control' sampling design conveys essentially the same amount of information as the whole cohort and already with two controls per case the loss of information with respect to studying the whole cohort is minor. Hence it becomes possible to perform the hormone determinations only on the blood of, say, 2,000 cases and 4,000 controls, namely a total of 6,000 women instead of on the blood of the several hundred thousand women in the EPIC cohort. This type of approach has become common in recent years in cohort studies involving biochemical or genetic tests on stored specimens of blood or other biological materials like urine and hair. The approach, usually called *case-control study within a cohort* or *nested case-control study*, may also be advantageously used in every situation in which assessing an exposure is very cumbersome or costly. This might be the case when investigating whether low doses of ionizing radiation cause cancer, which requires determining the amount of radiation received by each member of a large cohort of nuclear reactor workers in the course of their entire working life. This detailed evaluation can be limited to the cases of cancer and to a number of controls picked at random from among the workers rather than extended to everyone in the cohort.

Today's diseases arise from yesterday's causes

The sampling of a limited, but not too tiny, number of subjects out of a much larger cohort or population can be looked at from a different viewpoint. Ignoring the cohort for a moment, attention can be focused on the disease cases as the starting point of an investigation. This is what happens every day to doctors confronted with their patients. Again and again, keen doctors have been struck by the unusual occurrence of some events in the life experience of some of their patients providing the first hints to causes of the disease. For example, in the early 1960s an ear, nose, and throat specialist noted that as many as one-quarter of patients with cancer of the nasal cavities, a very rare disease, occurred in furniture workers, an infrequent type of exposure in the general population. This observation paved the way to subsequent epidemiological studies which showed that dusts produced in furniture and cabinet works can produce cancers of the nasal cavities, probably because the dust is loaded with several carcinogenic chemicals. Cancer of the nasal cavities and furniture making are both so rare that their repeated joint occurrence is unlikely to arise by chance. In ordinary circumstances, however, to judge whether such a joint occurrence is just coincidental requires some estimate of the frequency of the possible causal factor among the patients and in the general population from which they originate. Observing, as happened in the brief period of three years at a hospital in Boston, seven cases of cancer of the vagina in women as young as 15 to 22 immediately prompted an enquiry into the life experience of the patients extending into the pre-natal intrauterine period. Rather than focusing only on the patients, the investigators carefully selected for each case four controls: women born within five calendar days and in the same service (ward or private). Examination of the medical history of the patients' mothers during pregnancy found that all the mothers of the cases and none of the controls had been taking diethylstilbestrol, a synthetic oestrogen prescribed to prevent pregnancy loss in high-risk women. This *case-control* study provided strong evidence of a causal association between the drug and the cancer in daughters, explained on the basis of the alteration that it induced in the vaginal cells of the foetus that years later developed into a cancer. The use of the drug has since been proscribed.

Case-control studies were in fact widespread in epidemiology well before their use in the special situation where cases and controls are extracted from an actual study cohort. They can be regarded as a natural expansion of the enquiry a doctor makes the first time he or she sees a patient, asking not only about symptoms but also about the patient's health history, familial precedents, eating habits, occupation, and other elements which may possibly have a bearing on the present condition. In a case-control study, this procedure is carried out in a formalized way, using questionnaires focused on the exposure of interest to the investigator, and extending the enquiry to control subjects as well. The great advantage of this type of study is that it capitalizes on cases of disease which are occurring currently as a result of past causes – to be identified – rather than requiring, like a cohort study, a follow-up of subjects lasting years, waiting for the cases to occur.

Case-control studies have contributed knowledge to all areas of epidemiology and medicine. One example whose full relevance is now tangible are the seminal case-control studies tracking the causes of cervical cancer, today the second commonest cancer in women in developing countries. It had already been noted in the 19th century that this cancer was uncommon among nuns, suggesting that it was perhaps in some way connected with sexual activity. It then emerged from several case-control studies in the second half of the 20th century that the cancer was related to being married, particularly at an early age and to a high frequency of sexual intercourse. In one study, a frequency of intercourse of 15 times or more a month was 50% higher among the cancer cases than among the controls. In these studies, information on exposure (i.e. on frequency of intercourse) was collected, as very often in case-control studies, by interview and it could have been inaccurate; moreover, it was most likely that marriage and sexual intercourse were not directly relevant but reflected the action of some other unknown factor, probably infectious. The search for sexually transmitted micro-organisms started focusing in particular on several viruses, among which the human papilloma viruses (HPVs) were particularly suspect because they were known to produce benign tumour lesions in humans (warts) and malignant tumours in rabbits. Case-control studies in which the exposure was no longer the marital status nor the frequency of intercourse but the presence of the virus showed a strong association of some types of HPV with the cancer. The more specific and accurate was the laboratory method to ascertain the presence of the virus in cells of the uterine cervix, the stronger the association turned out to be, indicating that the virus, and not something else, was the real factor at play. Would this also mean that it was the cause of the cancer? It could in fact be that the cancer developed first and the virus was found only as a host boarding the cells once the cancer had begun. A case-control study is not a good instrument to solve this kind of 'who's first' question, because the presence of the virus (and in general of an exposure) is ascertained at the moment the disease is already established. Cohort studies showed that the infection with the virus preceded the cancer. Moreover, studies with newly developed vaccines demonstrated in a definitive way that the HPV viruses are the cause of cervical cancer and that blocking them prevents occurrence of the disease. Vaccination campaigns in young women are now in progress in several countries. Epidemiology has brought a crucial contribution to this major advance in public health, and case-control studies have been a pioneering component of it.

The four key features of case-control studies

1 The *selection of cases* is the starting point of case-control studies. Often, they are observed in hospital and the diagnosis can be accurate and if necessary refined, for example separating the different cellular types of lung cancer if one suspects that they may be influenced by different factors (exposures) to be investigated. Usually cases should have arisen very recently, i.e. they should be new or incident cases, for example of diabetes. If all cases of diabetes, whether they were diagnosed yesterday or ten years ago, are instead included in the study, it may happen that a factor emerging as different between cases and controls does in fact influence how long a diabetes patient survives rather than why a healthy subject becomes diabetic. These two features become

inextricable and the results of the study will become hard to interpret.

2 The *selection of controls* obeys the fundamental and rather obvious principle that they should come from the same *study population* as the cases. There are usually no problems when the population is an existing cohort already under investigation, as we have seen when discussing the case-control study within a cohort. A similar situation holds when the cases are, for example, all stomach cancers recorded in a year by a cancer registry covering a defined population, and controls are picked up at random from the population. The hurdle is that there will always be a proportion of selected controls who refuse to participate; they can be replaced by other people who consent to participate but in this way the controls are no longer rigorously representative of the population from which the cases come. When the latter is only vaguely defined, as when the cases are patients in a hospital, the problem of which population to sample to obtain controls may become very difficult. Taking as controls patients in the same hospital with diseases other than the one under study and not related to the factors under study is a widely adopted solution. It assumes that all kinds of patients reach the hospital for the same combination of reasons, medical, personal, administrative, or legal. This assumption may often be wrong as when, for example, the hospital has one highly specialized and reputed service for leukaemia, the disease under study, which receives patients from several regions while the other services of the hospital operate essentially on a local basis. In this situation, it is reasonable to select controls coming from the same area of residence of each case and it may be sensible to also match cases and controls for gender, age, interviewer, and calendar period of the interview. Going further and trying to find controls similar to the cases in other respects should be avoided. Not only is it difficult to find controls that match a case when the number of characteristics increases, but making cases and controls more and more similar makes the controls unrepresentative of their population of origin and destroys the

possibility of discovering differences in exposures between cases and controls, i.e. the very purpose of the study. The choice of controls is a major challenge for epidemiologists, requiring both experience – including mistakes – and specific knowledge of the local context of the study.

3 *Ascertaining exposure* very often involves interviewing cases and controls about a variety of factors to which they may have been exposed, ranging from smoking habits through diet to medical history, depending on the purpose of the study. The same interviewer interviews a case and his or her controls, in a random order and within a short period of time, to avoid subtle changes in the way questions are asked that may intervene with the passing of time (a case-control study usually lasts for months or a few years as necessary to obtain the required number of cases and controls). Structured questionnaires are the rule for the interview and interviewers undergo training sessions on how to use them and, more generally, on the approach to the subjects. Ideally the interviewers should not know whether the person they are talking to is a case or a control, as this would avoid bias in the way questions are formulated and answers recorded. This 'blind' condition is, however, seldom feasible in practice. In addition, the subjects themselves may remember incorrectly or report, consciously or unconsciously, past events and exposures. The extent to which this misreporting may be different for cases and controls produces a *recall bias* that distorts comparison. Similar problems affect telephone interviews and replies to self-administered questionnaires. Lesser difficulties arise when past exposures can be evaluated consulting written documents, for instance medical or employment records, although they may sometimes be incompletely or inaccurately filled in. Finally, an investigator may wish to explore the influence of a physiological factor like insulin on a disease such as colon cancer by measuring the blood levels of insulin in cases with colon cancer and controls without the disease; but who can guarantee that it is insulin influencing the disease rather than the other way round? Clearly

ascertaining exposure is a delicate exercise in a case-control setting.

4 By now you should have noted the basic difference between a case-control and a prospective study. The prospective study observes events in their natural course from causes to possible effects. Computing and comparing incidence rates or risks of chronic bronchitis in smokers and non-smokers seeks to answer the question: how often do smokers develop the disease compared to non-smokers? A case-control study observes the events in a reverse sequence, from effects to possible causes. It starts from the disease and seeks to answer the question: what proportion of people with chronic bronchitis have been smokers compared to people with no disease? No incidence rates or risks can be calculated from a case-control study as the number of smokers and non-smokers at risk of developing the disease is as a rule unknown; we only have two samples of people who actually developed or did not develop the disease but we know the frequency of smoking in both samples. Fortunately, a proper *data analysis* permits us to compute the ratio of the two risks, each of them remaining unknown. If this sounds surprising, consider for a moment the figures from a prospective study (not a case-control!) of a population of 10,000 people, of whom 2,515 turn out to be smokers and 7,485 non-smokers:

	Smokers	**Non-smokers**
Developed chronic bronchitis after three years of observation	25	15
Did not develop chronic bronchitis	2,490	7,470
Total population (10,000)	2,515	7,485

In three years, 25 smokers out of 2,515 developed chronic bronchitis, hence their risk is 25/2,515. Similarly, the risk for non-smokers is 15/7,485. The ratio of the two risks is (25/2,515) / (15/7,485) = (25/2,515) × (7,485/15) = 4.9, i.e. smokers have almost a fivefold probability of developing chronic bronchitis. We could get nearly the same result by replacing 2,515 (the number of smokers initially at risk of disease) with 2,490, the number that did not actually develop the disease by the end of the three years of observation. This replacement is justified by 2,490 being a reasonably close approximation to 2,515 and, similarly, 7,470 to 7,485. In general, the smaller the number of diseased people in relation to the population size, i.e. the disease risk during the period of observation, the better the approximation will be. And as any long period can be broken down into very tiny intervals, it will in principle be possible to make the risk within each interval as small as we please, rendering the approximation virtually perfect (a device you may come across under the intimidating name of 'incidence density sampling').

The new ratio, called the *odds ratio*, can now be computed as: (25/2,490)/(15/7,470) = (25/2,490) × (7,470/15) = 5.0, very close to 4.9.

Why go to the trouble of computing an odds ratio when the risk ratio is already available? Because the latter can, unlike the risk ratio, be calculated not only in a prospective study – as in the example – but also in a case-control study. For instance, a case-control study covering the same time span as our prospective study may have picked up from our population all 40 cases of bronchitis through hospital records and at random 160 controls without the disease, i.e. only 1.6 % of the 2,490 + 7,470 subjects with no disease. The new figures look like this:

	Smokers	**Non-smokers**
Cases with chronic bronchitis	25	15
Controls	40	120

The odds ratio is (25/40) / (15/120) = (25/40) × (120/15) = 5.0, exactly the same as before.

Herein lies the remarkable advantage of a case-control study: the possibility of estimating via the odds ratio computed from a comparatively small number of subjects the same ratio of risks that in a prospective setting would require following up a large population for years. This advantage offsets the limitations already discussed (notably in the choice of controls and in ascertainment of exposure) of case-control studies and explains their continuing popularity with epidemiologists. Problems notwithstanding, the case-control study is an epidemiological tool adaptable to all manners of circumstances and relatively rapid to implement. As such, it has been popular and is still currently used widely as a first-line study, when tackling a new health problem. When a group of people comes down with a serious gastrointestinal ailment after a festive dinner, the first thing an epidemiologist will do is to interview the sick people and then some healthy controls to ascertain the frequency with which individual food items served at the dinner were consumed by cases and controls. Hazardous items may in this way emerge and be identified and, hopefully, removed from the menu.

The boom in genetic case-control studies

Genes inherited from the parents are fixed characteristics of a living organism. They cannot be altered by the occurrence of a disease and they are not subject to recollection errors, unlike exposures ascertained by questioning cases and controls. For this reason, genes represent an ideal exposure to be measured accurately in case-control studies. Large series of cases, uniformly diagnosed, can be assembled from many clinical centres, providing adequate numbers for detecting associations between gene variants and disease. With the availability of techniques that permit testing a million 'single nucleotide polymorphisms' (SNPs), the gene variants already mentioned in Chapter 5, the current trend is to first throw the net wide and explore SNPs distributed over all 23 chromosomes. These studies are labelled 'GWAS', or Genome Wide Association Studies, and after the first phase are followed by confirmatory phases to check that the associations found in the first phase are not false positive results arising simply by chance. Several GWAS studies are in progress and many more are starting. The first results of one large study of 14,000 cases of seven common diseases and 3,000 controls has identified more than 20 associations, involving a mental disorder, coronary artery disease, type 1 and type 2 diabetes, an intestinal inflammatory disease, and rheumatoid arthritis.

Confirmed associations open the way to the investigation of the physiological mechanisms leading from the gene variant to the disease, a task beyond the scope of ordinary case-control studies. In principle, blood could be taken from cases and controls and biochemical studies carried out to probe these mechanisms. However, the presence of the disease makes the meaning of any physiological finding questionable: would it really represent a step leading to the disease or instead be a consequence of the disease itself? Only case-control studies conducted within cohorts where blood was collected and stored before the disease occurred, like the EPIC or the British Biobank cohorts, are free of this problem. Laboratory studies on experimental animals and on cells, including fresh white blood cells from human volunteers, complement these epidemiology based studies on the physiological paths linking genes to disease. Understanding these paths also helps to clarify the role of the external factors at play. Drugs and other means (e.g. changes in diet) that can interfere with the paths and prevent disease development are the ultimate objective of this research.

Chapter 8
Mapping health and disease

Space, time, and individuals

Intervention studies, randomized or non-randomized, and observational studies (cohort and case-control) form the core of epidemiology. As they aim to test hypotheses about causal relationships between exposures and effects, they are often collectively called *analytical studies* (cross-sectional and correlation studies, of which more later on in this chapter, also belong to the group). Analytical studies are generally both preceded and followed by *descriptive studies* of how health and disease, as measured by rates of deaths, new cases of disease, or hospital admissions, are distributed in space by geographical area, in time by week or month or year, and in categories of people of different age, gender, and socio-economic status. Observing a disease distribution in space, time, and categories of people provides useful indications of which factors need to be explored in depth through analytical studies as possible determinants of the distribution. Visually friendly tools, like graphs and maps (sometimes collected in atlases), convey a pictorial view of disease burden and evolution, as in the examples of Figures 9 to 12. They facilitate the examination of descriptive data and the generation of causal hypotheses.

Cholera made headlines in 2008 when a lethal epidemic hit Zimbabwe, but in the 19th century it had often ravaged Europe, producing waves of high mortality, particularly among the poorest sections of the population living in squalid conditions. From foci in India, it spread to Europe, and Figure 9, an early example (1832) of a health map, illustrates its progression westward.

Today, cholera has practically disappeared from Europe while cardiovascular diseases head the league of causes of mortality. In particular, death rates from heart attacks, mapped in Figure 10, tend to be markedly higher in northeast than in southwest Europe.

Sixty years ago, the marked difference in the occurrence of heart attacks between southern Europe and other regions, especially the United States, prompted American investigators to develop a comparative cohort study in seven countries with very different rates (Finland, Greece, Italy, Japan, the Netherlands, the United States, Yugoslavia). Together with other cohorts, especially the Framingham study, this 'Seven Country study', follow-up of which has continued until recently, has provided essential information to establish high cholesterol, tobacco smoking, and high blood pressure as three major determinants of heart attacks.

Diseases vary both in the short and long term. Figure 11 depicts the rise and fall of an outbreak of a viral disease, mumps, communicable from person to person through airborne droplets or saliva: it was a small (37 cases), self-limiting, and non-lethal outbreak localized particularly in a school. Epidemic curves are not only useful as visual summaries of past epidemics. When constructed day by day or week by week while an epidemic is in progress, they allow, combined with information on the mechanism of transmission of the disease, the building of mathematical models, deterministic or probabilistic, predicting the likely evolution of the disease.

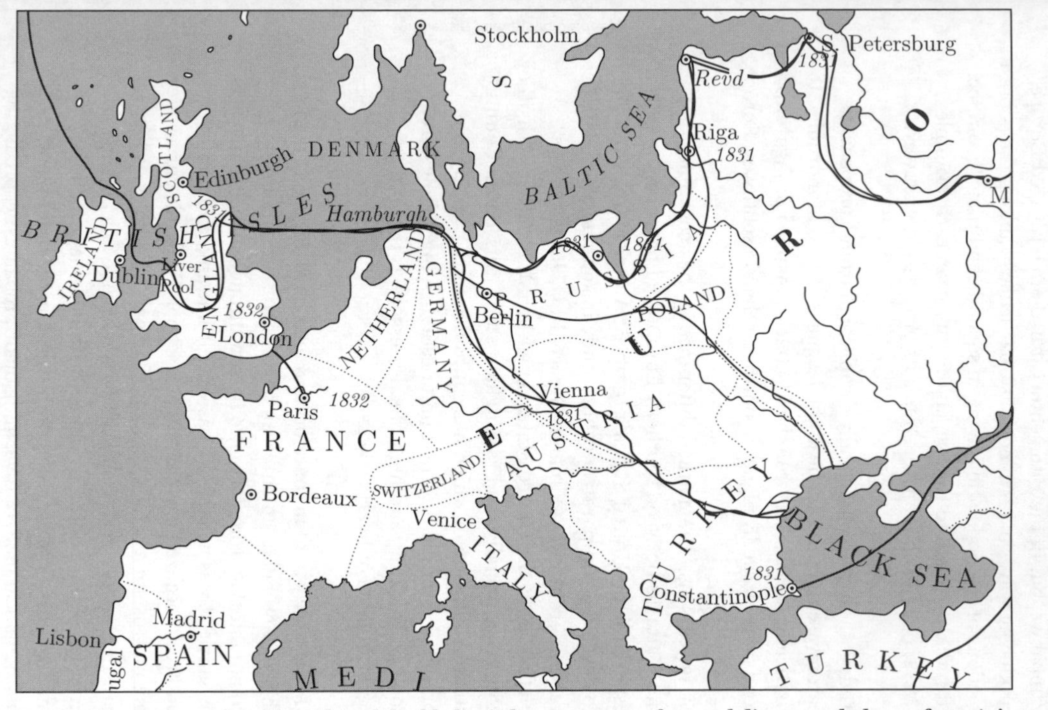

9. An 1832 disease map sketching (dotted double line) the movement of a novel disease – cholera – from Asia to Western Europe and England

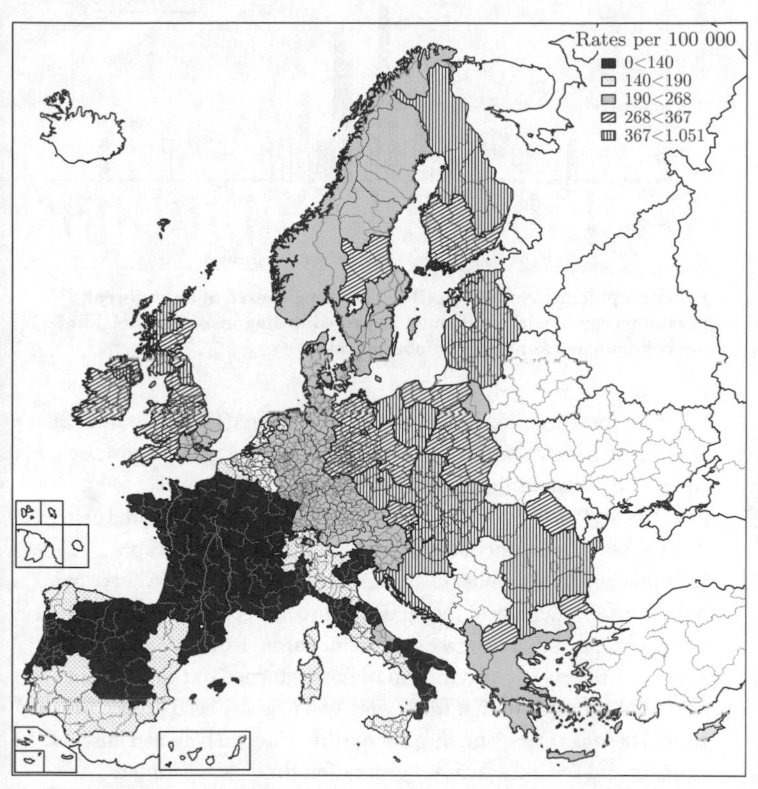

10. Mortality rates from heart attacks in men aged 45–74 years in Europe

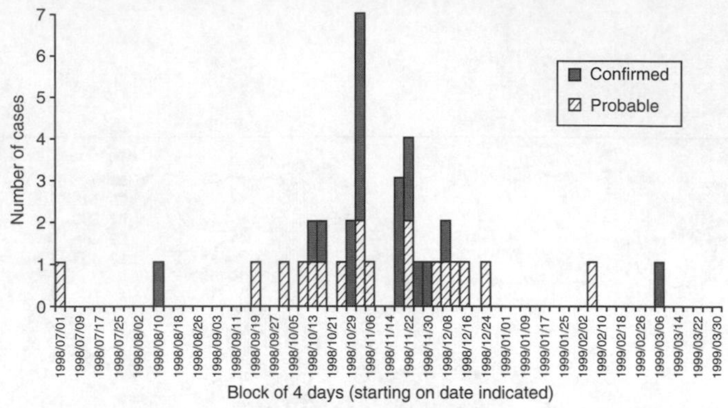

11. The 'epidemic curve' describing the time course of an outbreak of mumps cases, with confirmed or probable diagnosis. The height of the columns measures the number of cases

Figure 12 portrays the development of the new A(H1/N1) influenza among the nearly 1,600 residents of the La Gloria village in Mexico, where the disease, initially labelled as 'swine flu', was first recognized. The two continuous bell-shaped curves, calculated using two very similar mathematical models, follow well the graph (columns) of daily number of cases. From the equation of a curve two important coefficients of the epidemic process could be estimated. The average number of new cases arising through direct contact with a primary flu case ('reproduction number') turned out to be about 1.6, roughly meaning that from every two primary cases, three secondary ones arise; and the average time interval between onset of primary and secondary cases ('generation time') was estimated at about 2 days. These coefficients are key elements when attempting to project how widely and how fast an epidemic can develop.

Descriptive studies not only stimulate and guide the development of analytical epidemiological studies but are also an ultimate check that the results of the latter 'make sense'. If tobacco smoking is an important cause of lung cancer, the pattern of lung cancer rates by geographical area and over a period of years should reflect, or at least

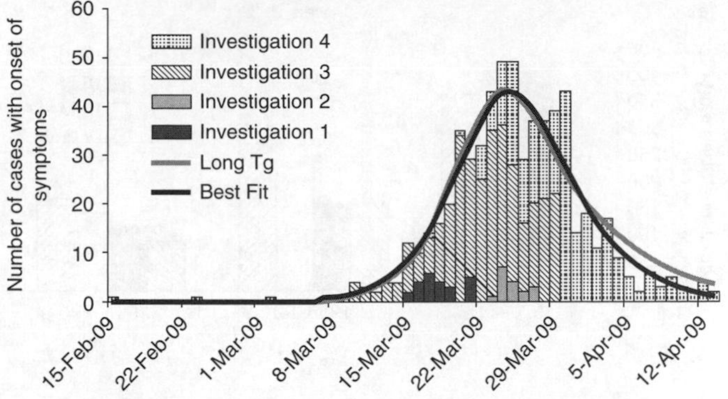

12. The 'epidemic curve' of the outbreak of the new A(H1/N1) influenza in the village of La Gloria, state of Veracruz, Mexico, 2009

be compatible with, the pattern of tobacco consumption, as has in fact been found again and again in many countries. And if effective measures of prevention have been taken, for instance reducing tobacco consumption or removing a pollutant or treating a disease, they should be reflected in a change in the rates of the disease.

Figure 13 demonstrates the dual role of descriptive statistics. Preventive measures and improved treatment in fact show up in the halving of the risk of heart attacks between the late 1970s and the late 1990s; at the same time, the persistent difference between higher and lower social classes is a stimulus for new research.

Sources of data

The description of health and disease in populations relies on data that are collected on an ongoing and systematic basis or through special enquiries. In principle, all countries in the world (192 are members of the World Health Organization) have a system of records of basic life events: births, deaths, and causes of deaths. The organization and, more importantly, the coverage and quality

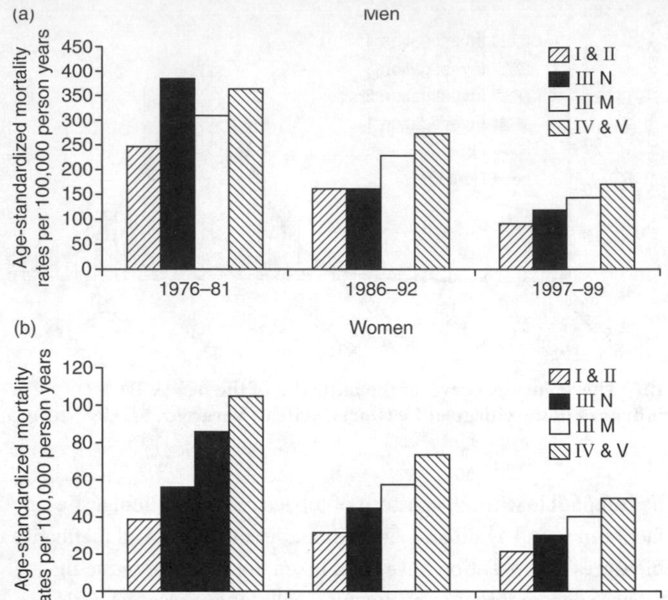

13. In England and Wales, the risk of dying from a heart attack, measured by the height of the rectangles, has almost halved in the last quarter of the 20th century but continues to be higher for people of less favourable socio-economic positions (classes IV and V, and III M) than for the better off (classes I and II, and III N)

of the data collected are very variable. Only 20% of the world's population living in 75 countries, mostly economically developed, is in fact covered by cause-of-death statistics judged (for instance in respect to accuracy, completeness, and other requirements) as high or medium-high quality. For as many as 25% of the world population, WHO does not receive any data on cause of death. Several years, from three to ten or more, may be needed for cause of death to be reported to WHO and made available for international comparisons. As to births, 36% go unregistered, with vast differences between countries, from 2% in industrialized countries to 71% in the very least developed. In the decade 1995–2004, only 30% of the six billion world population lived in countries with complete registration of births and deaths. This percentage had not changed much from the 27% figure of the period 1965–74 (when the world population was less than 4 billion).

Morbidity statistics are disease-oriented, and range from hospital discharge records, in principle available wherever a hospital exists but in practice of vastly variable quality, to registries intended to cover all cases of a disease, or of a group of diseases, occurring within a population. In selected and limited areas of a number of developed countries, registries are operational for malformations, myocardial infarctions, diabetes, stroke, and other conditions. Cancer or, better, cancers (because the heading embraces several hundred different diseases), is the condition best covered. Cancer registries started in the 1930s in North America and the first nationwide registry was established in Denmark in 1942. By the end of the last century, there were close to 200 good-quality cancer registries, mostly local or regional, in 57 countries.

Because of the danger of contagion, several infectious diseases have been the object of compulsory and rapid notification at national level since the late 19th century. Today, cases of diseases such as smallpox, SARS, poliomyelitis, and cholera fall within the larger scope of the 'International Health Regulations' and also require notification to the World Health Organization. Surveillance systems of communicable diseases have evolved in promptness and coverage, yet even the best systems based on doctors' diagnoses can hardly report a rising epidemic in less than one or two weeks. Recently, and somewhat surprisingly, just counting an increasing number of daily queries on influenza in Google has proved capable of detecting the rise of the disease in just one or two days. This simple and cheap approach might also work for other epidemic diseases in areas with a large population of Web users. An accurate estimate of the propagation and severity of a potentially fatal disease demands, however, a complete enumeration both of cases and of deaths. When many mild cases are not recorded, as it may be for the A(H1/N1) influenza, the extent and speed of the epidemic is underestimated and the *fatality rate*, i.e. the ratio of deaths to cases in a time interval, is overestimated (as deaths are less likely to go unrecorded).

Friendly figures and hidden fallacies

The map of heart attacks throughout Europe (Figure 10) may suggest among others the hypothesis that the disease distribution is related to some foods, a possibility which can be explored by correlating the rates of heart attacks in each European country (or even within smaller areas) with the average per capita consumption of several foods. Both the figures for heart attacks and for food consumption can be gathered easily from published statistics, making the exercise fast and friendly. If we had only two countries, one with a high consumption of, say, milk and the other with a low consumption, we could simply compute, as we have learned from Chapter 4, a rate ratio. A ratio different from 1 (equality of rates) would tell (if statistically significant) that there is an association or correlation between the occurrence of heart attacks and the consumption of milk. Here, however, we have not two but several countries, and correspondingly several rates and differing levels of milk consumption; fortunately, the method of studying their correlation is just an extension of the rate ratio. If a correlation is indeed found, we should guard against inferring that milk consumption is a determinant of heart attacks. Not only do we have to take into account the possibility of confounding and bias encountered when interpreting associations in general, but here the association, called an *ecological association*, is at the level of geographical units, i.e. countries, not at the level of individuals, as in case-control and cohort studies. In these, the consumption of milk and the health status (with or without heart attack) would have been measured and be known for each person, while in the correlation exercise all that is known is the rate for each country and the average consumption of milk (derived, for example, from sales figures). No one knows whether within each country the individuals who develop a heart attack are those who also consume more milk and the observed correlation could be an artefact. Falsely believing that it is real would result in an *ecological fallacy*. As is often heard, and as epidemiologists, contrary to what is also often heard, know perfectly well 'correlation is not causation'.

Things, however, are even more complex as an opposite fallacy may be at work. Imagine two areas in one of which nobody smokes while in the other everybody smokes the same amount from the age of 15. The latter would have a much higher rate of lung cancer than the former, yet a study measuring smoking habits for each individual would be unable to detect any difference in lung cancer risk associated with smoking within each area. Only comparison of the two areas would reveal that in these circumstances smoking is a determinant of lung cancer but only at the population (area) level. To look only at the individual level may lead to an *atomistic fallacy*. Everything that has been said about geographical units applies also to time units, for example to correlations of concentrations of air pollutants during successive weeks and hospital admission rates for respiratory disease in the same weeks.

Cross-sectional surveys

Detailed information on health is gathered by special surveys of samples of a population, in which questions about health are asked or a health examination is carried out, or both. As in correctly conducted opinion polls, representative samples can be obtained by first subdividing the population by key criteria, typically gender, age, place of residence, and then extracting at random within each subdivision or 'stratum' a number of subjects to be included in the survey. All data collected refer, as in population censuses, to a fixed point in time (calendar date) even if the actual duration may span several days or weeks. Some surveys may be repeated regularly to monitor trends in health. A major periodical survey is the US National Health and Nutrition Examination Survey. It was first conducted in the period 1971–75 on a nationwide random sample of more than 30,000 subjects and included an interview focused on diet and a medical examination. The survey was repeated in 1976–80 and in 1997–8. Since 1999, it has become an ongoing biennial survey including an enlarged and variable number of interview, medical examination, and laboratory test items.

While it is valuable to document in detail the health of a community and its changes in time, these surveys are usually less useful as tools to search for causes of disease. For example, blood pressure measurements and an electrocardiogram can be taken during the survey, and some electrocardiogram anomalies may be found to be more frequent among people with high blood pressure than among people with normal blood pressure. However, as both electrocardiogram and blood pressure were assessed at the same time, it is impossible to say which anomaly started first and can be a cause, direct or indirect, of the other. Indeed, they may both have begun at about the same time as the result of another common factor, such as tobacco smoking. All surveys of this type that collect data only once at a fixed point in time (*cross-sectional studies*) suffer from this shortcoming. Surveys of the same populations repeated at different dates but, as is often the case, on a different sample of people are not free of this limitation.

The burden of diseases

Another minefield, essential for the establishment of public health priorities, is the determination of the burden of different diseases due to different factors in a region or nation or even worldwide. In its simplest form, this may start with a frequently asked question of the type: what percentage of, for example, all cancers is due, say, to environment? Three main problems prevent a single answer. First, the definition of environment may cover all factors external to the body (sunlight, pollutants in air and water, tobacco smoke, foods, etc.) or it may be restricted to some of them, like pollutants in place of residence and occupation: the percentages will vary depending on the definition. A second reason is that these percentages obviously depend on how many people are exposed to the different components of the environment: if many smoke, the percentage of cancers due to environment, and to smoke in particular, is high; if few smoke, it is low. How many people smoke (and how much) may be relatively easy to determine, but there is usually much more uncertainty on how many people are exposed, for example, to carcinogenic air pollutants; moreover, for both exposures the numbers of exposed individuals vary from place to place, and percentages calculated for large countries or continents or the entire world hide these substantial variations as well as the uncertainty in the evaluation of the numbers of exposed people.

Finally, even accurate percentages specific to a single place (e.g. a town) have the puzzling feature that they cannot be added up, as their total may exceed 100%, i.e. more than the total of cancer cases! In fact, if we knew all causes of cancer perfectly – which is far from being the case today – there would be a lot of double counting, as many cancers are due to the joint action of two or more causes, genetic and environmental. As we have seen in Chapter 5, occupational exposure to asbestos and tobacco smoking both independently increase the risk of lung cancer, but their combination further multiplies the risk for asbestos workers who smoke. It is correct to attribute the percentage of cancers due to this combined action, say 5% of all lung cancers, once to asbestos and once to smoking (because without either of the two exposures these cancers would have not occurred), but it is not correct to sum the corresponding percentages, 5% + 5%, because they refer to the same cancers.

With all these reservations, it should not be surprising if today one cannot be more precise than saying that on the grand scale of the whole world approximately one-third of cancer is attributable to environmental factors. Tobacco smoking accounts for at least 20%, alcoholic drinks for some 5%, infectious agents for at least 10% with higher percentages in developing countries, and occupational and environmental carcinogens for fractions variable from less than 1% to some 10%.

These percentages are a simplistic representation of the actual impact of a factor on the health of a population. The same percentage may reflect impacts of very different severity depending on whether the cancers affect young or old people or whether they are successfully treatable (and how and for how long) or not. These elements are taken into account in sophisticated analyses, developed in the last two decades, of the *burden of disease* in local, national, or world populations. Often, the results of burden of disease analyses are expressed as number of DALYs (disability-adjusted life years) lost due to a cause. One DALY corresponds to the loss of one year of life free of disability: hence the DALY unit of measurement incorporates both the loss of years of life, because of death, and the loss of quality of life, because of disability.

Chapter 9
From epidemiology to medicine, prevention, and public health

Working for the health of all

Epidemiology is at heart a field of applied research with the improvement of the health of all as the key aim. As such, epidemiology is an essential component of all public health activities that implement the organized efforts of society to promote, protect, and restore health.

This concept of public health has no relation to how societal efforts to improve health are or should be organized; it does, however, imply that some kind of explicit organization should exist, rather than just dispersed and uncoordinated initiatives, for society to successfully tackle health problems.

As shown in Figure 14, three broad activities contribute to people's health. In clinical medicine, doctors and other health personnel deal individually with each patient. They provide preventive measures such as drugs to control high cholesterol or elevated blood pressure, or deliver advice and psychological support to stop smoking. They intervene to diagnose, treat, and when possible cure, diseases with procedures ranging from the simple prescription of an antibiotic to a complex liver or heart transplant. Finally, they offer individual rehabilitation to people with disabling diseases.

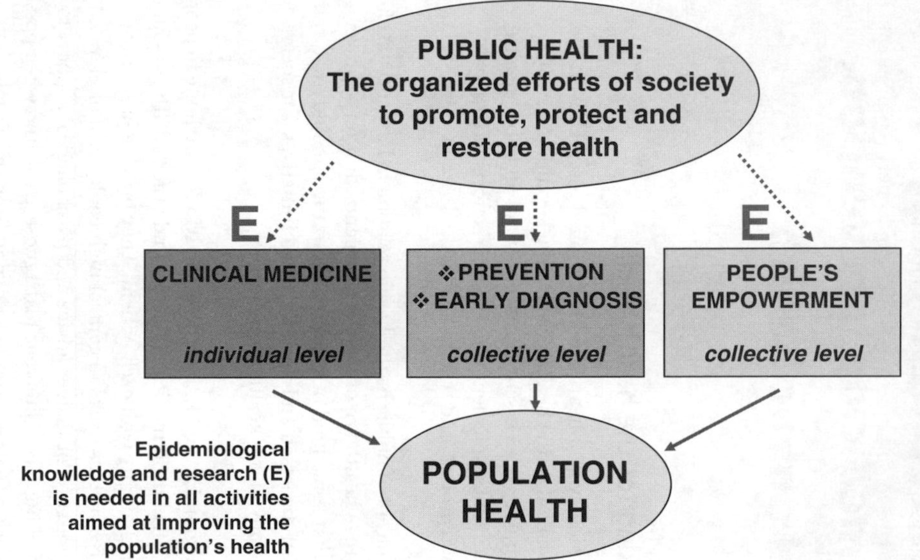

14. Public health activities

Prevention and early diagnosis at the population level form the second field of activity. Prevention addresses the root causes of disease, environmental or genetic. It embraces a vast array of regulations spanning control of pollutants in air, water, and the workplace, to traffic speed limits and safety requirements in home appliances. It includes compulsory and optional vaccination programmes as well as campaigns to foster healthy diet and behaviour. When it targets genetic causes of diseases, for example the screening of all newborns for genetic defects, primary prevention uses medical diagnostic tools, as do organized programmes of early diagnosis and treatment of diseases. These have proved effective and are operational in many countries for a limited number of high-impact diseases such as cancers of the uterine cervix and of the breast.

The third activity consists in the empowerment of people to exercise responsibility for their health through adoption of health-promoting habits and participation in the decision processes that shape health policies. The latter in turn may reinforce or inhibit people's empowerment, the development of which depends on formal and informal education and on updated and accurate information.

Public health also coordinates these activities in relation to other societal actions, external to the health system, which strongly influence health, for example income and housing policies. In the coordination process, public health administrators and policy makers usually demand that the benefits and adverse effects of proposed policies be subject to economic analysis, in which epidemiologists play a specific role jointly with other specialists.

Channelling the research results into practice, whether in clinical medicine, in population prevention, or for people's empowerment, requires as a first step the aggregation of the results of multiple studies to consolidate the total evidence available on a specific question, for example whether vitamin C protects against cancer in humans. This is done by critically reviewing the studies' reports, comparing methods and results, and drawing a general 'best' answer to the question at hand. In the last two decades, the approach and methods used in a review, previously entirely left to the reviewer's discretion, have been refined and made more objective and rigorous under the heading of *systematic reviews*.

Systematic reviews, with and without meta-analysis

A systematic review is a review carried out using a systematic approach to minimize bias and random errors, a process which is explicitly documented in the methods section of the review itself. It usually offers a more objective appraisal of the available evidence than traditional reviews, conducted as narrative commentaries on the studies. In a systematic review, each study is scrutinized to assess its quality in respect of a number of criteria fixed in advance, e.g. how well the population is defined, whether the study responses were assessed blindly or not, and so on. This makes it possible to consider separately studies judged of higher and lower quality, rather than all of them together, and see whether the results of the lower-quality studies point in the same direction (e.g. towards a reduction or an increase in risk) as the higher-quality ones. Broadly consistent results can be combined in a statistical analysis, a *meta-analysis*, to provide a single summary estimate of risk. This analysis, in which each study is given a 'weight' proportional to the number of disease cases it contributes, may cause a clear-cut result to emerge, while the individual studies, particularly if small in size, may each present a result statistically non-significant that is difficult to interpret.

Combining studies often permits the evaluation of rare events, too few of which occur in a single study. A typical case is that of side effects of new drugs, which occur infrequently, say once in a thousand treated patients. However, if a side effect is serious, for instance a major heart problem, it will have considerable impact when the drug is put on the market and used by hundreds of thousands or millions of people. Yet such an effect will be hard to detect in a randomized experiment of a size of, say, a few hundred subjects, which would be more than adequate to measure a much more frequent therapeutic effect. It is only by combining all available data from different randomized experiments that a sufficiently large number of patients is reached to allow the adverse event to become detectable. A telling example is Rofecoxib, a drug commercialized in 1999 as an anti-inflammatory remedy for rheumatic and muscular disorders. It was withdrawn from the market by the manufacturer in September 2004 on account of an increased risk of heart attacks, when an estimated 80 million people had already used it. However, if the manufacturer or the drug licensing authorities had conducted a timely meta-analysis, they would have detected the increased risk more than three years earlier, in 2000, as Figure 15 clearly shows (the meta-analysis of this figure was retrospectively performed in 2004 by independent academic epidemiologists).

Systematic reviews complemented by meta-analyses of randomized controlled trials are most valuable for clinical medicine. They have helped to develop the continuously evolving body of *evidence-based medicine* which guides doctors' everyday practice. They have also helped to put the evidence from randomized preventive trials carried out in populations on a firm basis, for example the prevention of myocardial infarction with cholesterol-lowering drugs.

Meta-analyses have also been extended to observational epidemiology studies directly relevant to public health. Combining results from observational studies in which confounding factors and biases have usually been dealt with in a different way in each

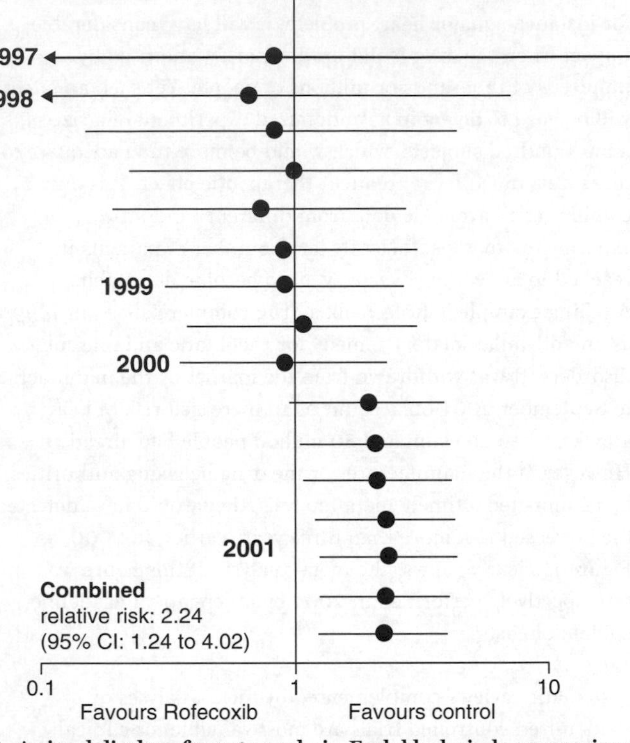

15. A visual display of a meta-analysis. Each black circle summarizes the risk of myocardial infarction from all randomized studies available till the beginning of each year among people treated with Rofecoxib relative to the risk among people treated with a control drug

study in a statistical analysis is, however, problematic. As we know from Chapter 5, in randomized controlled trials bias and confounding are prevented by randomization and do not impinge on a meta-analysis, a condition that does not apply to observational studies. For these studies, systematic reviews are in any case necessary while the worth of meta-analyses has to be assessed case by case.

Clinical medicine

Systematic reviews form an important part of clinical epidemiology, but more generally the quantitative and probabilistic traits of epidemiology pervade clinical medicine. It is common to find today in standard textbooks of medicine references to 'NNTs' and schemes of 'diagnostic decision trees'. Comparing treatment options is helped by computing the NNT, or *number needed to treat*. In severe hypertensive subjects, the risk of a major adverse outcome (such as death or stroke) in the coming three years may be as high as 20%. A treatment may, however, reduce it to 15%. The risk reduction obtained with the treatment is $20 - 15 = 5\%$, which means that out of 100 subjects treated, 5 avoid the major adverse outcome they would have otherwise suffered. This is the same as saying that for one subject to avoid a major adverse event, the number needing treatment is $100/5 = 20$. Should a new treatment reduce the risk to 4%, it would be necessary to treat only $6 \sim= 100 / (20 - 4)$ patients to avoid one adverse event. Comparing the number of people who need to be treated for the two treatments, 20 against 6, conveys tangible information on the merits of the two treatments, the second being clearly superior (provided all other aspects are the same, for instance the frequency of side effects, but these can be dealt with in terms similar to NNT).

A *diagnostic decision tree* is designed to assist the physician in formulating a diagnosis. If a young man presents with a sudden vague but aching and recurrent pain in the left chest, one diagnostic possibility is coronary artery disease, the narrowing of the coronary arteries that supply blood to the heart. Given the young age of the patient and the absence of any other sign, this condition appears *a priori* unlikely, but being very serious it could be disastrous to miss it. The patient can thus undergo an exercise stress test whereby his electrocardiogram is monitored during controlled physical effort. A negative test would be reassuring; unfortunately the test is not perfect and sometimes it turns out falsely negative even in presence of the disease, in the same way that it can be falsely positive in its absence. If narrative terms like '*a priori* unlikely', 'sometimes falsely positive', 'sometimes falsely negative' are replaced with figures of probabilities (derived from specific studies), a map, or decision tree, can be built of all possible courses of diagnostic actions. One course may be to dismiss straight away the diagnosis of coronary artery disease because the type of pain found in an otherwise healthy and young man makes the diagnosis less than 5% probable. The alternative course is to proceed to the stress test knowing, however, that it has a 30% probability of false negative results (i.e. it has a *sensitivity* of 100 − 30 = 70%) and a 10% probability of false positive results (i.e. it has a *specificity* of 100 − 10 = 90%). Combining these figures makes it possible to calculate the probability, or *predictive power*, that each alternative will correctly identify the disease if present or dismiss it if absent. A comparison of these probabilities, and of the penalties involved in a wrong diagnosis, helps the physician to analyse the diagnostic process, which often involves not just one but many possible tests, and to choose an optimal diagnostic strategy (these calculations are based on *Bayes' theorem*, a fundamental tool for drawing inferences of probabilistic nature from empirical observations, established as early as the mid-18th century by the Reverend Thomas Bayes).

Prevention and early diagnosis

In a strict technical sense, 'prevention' denotes the activities aimed at directly modifying the root determinants of disease, which fall only into two broad categories: genes and environment, or in more archaic wording 'nature and nurture'. Early diagnosis, on the other hand, aims at detecting and treating diseases before they become manifest through symptoms. These two neatly separated activities, both organized at the level of the whole population, have, however, a major bridge in the diagnosis of host risk factors, like high blood cholesterol or high blood pressure, that are not yet 'diseases' but increase the chance of disease occurrence; on the one side, the host risk factors share this property with a person's genes predisposing to disease, while on the other they are themselves the result, like early disease, of a complex interplay of genes and environment.

Some early disease diagnosis tests are carried out as 'opportunistic screening tests' by individual doctors when they examine a patient: for instance, the PSA test for prostate cancer discussed in Chapter 5 has become, rightly or wrongly, popular in several developed countries even in the absence of firm evidence of net benefit. Only screenings for which this evidence exists do, however, qualify for systematic adoption in the population in the form of 'organized screening programmes', such as those for colon cancer or for cervical and breast cancer in women, now implemented on a substantial scale in many countries. Screening programmes aimed at early diagnosis in apparently healthy populations are evaluated in the same ways as the diagnostic procedures in symptomatic patients previously discussed. Programmes for different diseases can be compared or different alternatives of a programme, for instance screening for cervical cancer using either the cytological 'Pap test' or the assay detecting the human papilloma virus. For this purpose, indexes such as the predictive power and the *number needed to screen* (NNS) are calculated. The latter is closely similar to the number needed to treat (NNT) and tells how many subjects one needs to test in order to avoid one death or other major adverse event within a period of time. It depends not only, as NNT does, from the probability that a treatment successfully avoids death but also from the probability that an apparently healthy subject turns out to have the disease without symptoms. NNS are usually in the range from several hundreds to, more often, several thousands.

Screening for host factors, genetic or acquired, that may predispose to a disease stands on the basic assumption that subjects who will develop the disease can be distinguished from subjects who will not, so that any preventive intervention, for example a change in diet, can be concentrated on the former (should the distinction prove impossible, there would be no point in screening and any intervention would simply need to be applied to everybody). Looking closely at one of these risk factors, blood cholesterol, throws light on how far the basic assumption is justified and illustrates at the same time some general principles of prevention, taken in the wide and generic sense of any measure able to prevent at any point the progression from health to disease and death.

Today, few will be surprised if a heavy smoker comes down with lung cancer. Many may be surprised, however, if told that avoiding heavy smoking will not wipe out the burden of lung cancer in the population because a substantial number of cases occur in fact in people who regularly smoke only moderately. What is true for smoking holds even more for blood cholesterol, as this set of figures shows:

Categories of cholesterol levels in millimoles per litre	**Percentage of the population**	**Percentage of deaths from heart attacks in each category**
0.0 – 3.9	8	-
4.0 – 4.4	13	4
4.5 – 4.9	18	8
5.0 – 5.4	22	17
5.5 – 5.9	17	22
6.0 – 6.4	11	19
6.5 – 6.9	6	13
7.0 – 7.4	3	9
7.5 – 8.0	2	8

People with frankly anomalous cholesterol levels, say above 6.5 millimoles per litre, represent $6+3+2=11\%$ of the population in which it has been found that $13+9+8=30\%$ of the deaths from heart attacks occur (in case you feel more comfortable with milligrams per 100 millilitres, 6.5 millimoles is about 250 milligrams). Intervening on this 'high-risk' fraction of the population, about one-tenth of the total, would prevent – assuming an intervention that is 100% effective – just one-third of the deaths, leaving untouched the other two-thirds. Why these disappointing results? Because the risk is not concentrated solely in people 'at high risk', with cholesterol levels above 6.5 millimoles, but involves everybody to some degree. As cholesterol levels increase over the very lowest levels (category 0–3.9), the risk of disease increases by small increments, with no abrupt jumps.

As a consequence, the many people with only modest elevations in cholesterol who are also at a modestly increased risk produce more cases of heart attacks than the minority of people at high risk. This 'paradox of prevention' implies that the bulk of cases could be prevented by moderately reducing the cholesterol level, hence the risk, of everybody. Abating cholesterol only in people with high levels is certainly beneficial to them but cannot do the public health job of preventing the mass of cases in the population. Many disease determinants have been found to increase the risk of some diseases in a smooth, continuous way like cholesterol, for example blood pressure for heart attacks, hydraulic pressure in the eye for glaucoma, or alcohol consumption for cancer of the oesophagus or liver cirrhosis.

The graded distribution over the whole population of risk generated by these determinants, rather than its exclusive concentration in some groups, stresses their role as population disease determinants, discussed in Chapter 4 in contrast to individual determinants. The susceptibility of each person, rooted in their genetic make-up, plays – as does chance – a role in determining who becomes diseased, but the number affected will depend to a major extent on the population determinants. For example, there are no known populations with a high frequency of heart attacks without also an average (over the whole population) high level of cholesterol. The next question then becomes: why do population determinants differ from one population to another? Cholesterol level is diet dependent and, like alcohol consumption, is conditioned by available foods (or alcoholic drinks), traditional tastes, and behaviour influenced by marketing and by economic constraints. For infectious diseases, the proportion of people vaccinated is a typical population determinant of how often a disease will occur, because vaccinated people do not fall ill and at the same time they interrupt the chain of transmission of the contagion.

For most diseases, multiple, rather than single, determinants are recognized. For example, blood cholesterol level, blood pressure, tobacco smoking, diabetes, and obesity are main population determinants of heart attacks. Interventions acting in turn on these determinants aim at promoting healthy habits, behaviours, foods, and to limit the availability of harmful products. This population strategy of prevention, based on a variable mix of incentives, education, and regulation, is beneficial to everybody, whatever one's known or unknown susceptibility or level of risk. It can be complemented by specific preventive actions, often involving the use of drugs (e.g. to lower cholesterol or blood pressure) for people known to be at definitely high risk. Recently the idea has dawned that a combination in a single pill ('polypill') of low doses of several drugs controlling cholesterol level, blood pressure, and blood clotting propensity could be used in a population prevention strategy by offering it to most or all middle-aged and older people. Whether this is an effective, safe, and realistic possibility remains to be explored. The general principle is that before being launched on a grand scale, a preventive measure must have been clearly shown to work. This involves research covering a large number (Figure 16) of disease determinants, from proximate biological and genetic factors, to personal behaviour

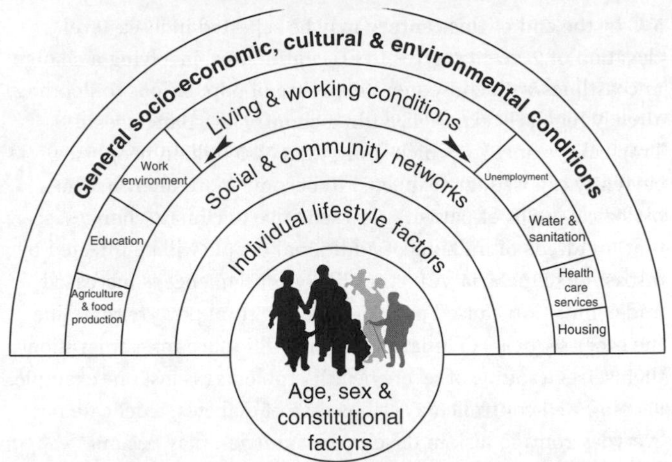

16. Health and disease are shaped by a wide range of determinants, from social, economic, and political conditions or climatic changes to individual lifestyle and genetic factors

traits, and to the 'determinants of the determinants' operating at the level of the social or of the global environment.

Attention to the global environment has markedly increased in recent years. Localized 'heat waves' have caused clearly documented excesses of mortality and fluctuations in urban air pollutants, especially fine particulates, which have been shown to increase hospital admissions for respiratory and cardiovascular ailments and to precipitate deaths from a variety of causes. Protocols to prevent these adverse effects affecting in particular vulnerable, already sick people have been put in place in a number of countries.

In contrast to these meteorological episodes, the health consequences of the foreseen global climatic change are a completely new chapter for epidemiological investigation. A likely temperature increase of anything between 2°C and

5°C by the end of this century may be reflected in a sea-level elevation of 20 centimetres to 60 centimetres, involving a change in coastlines with consequent exposure of populations to flooding, already regularly experienced in a country like Bangladesh. Tropical cyclones, to which more than 300 million people are currently exposed, are expected to become more intense. The biological cycles of parasites are sensitive to climate changes, so that hundreds of millions of additional people will be infected by diseases like malaria. A further likely consequence is increased under-nutrition caused by droughts and rural poverty that, like the other sequels of climatic change, will induce mass migrations, themselves a source of severe health problems (as just one example, keeping well controlled a serious case of diabetes, a delicate but everyday routine task in developed countries, may become hopeless in a moving refugee population). Today, these effects can be identified but their probable impact on health (currently quite modest) remains to be quantified through research that combines available epidemiological data, for example on malaria in different regions, with models simulating how the disease may evolve under various hypotheses of temperature and other environmental changes.

Empowering people

In an equal rights society, every citizen ought to be empowered to take part in decisions affecting her or his health and, through democratic processes (on which more in Chapter 10), in deliberations concerning the health of the population. This can come about through information, conditioning, or education. There are innumerable sources of information: newspapers, magazines, books, television, and, most prominently, the Internet. There are close to 100,000 sites on the Web dealing with health matters and a major issue is the accuracy of the information. Studies are being done to measure the risk of encountering inaccurate sources, and private and public accreditation systems are being developed.

Almost everybody with access to the Web searches it occasionally or regularly on health, usually in relation to actual or possible health problems. Texts found for this reason or for curiosity or cultural interest need to be interpreted in the light of two considerations. First, most descriptions are inherently probabilistic, based as they must be on risks and rates of success of a preventive measure or of a treatment, or rates and risks of harm from side effects of a drug, from an unhealthy food, or from smoking marijuana, say. Second, the presentation is usually influenced by who is providing the information and for what declared or implicit purpose. It may be impartial and strictly to the point or framed in a wider educational context (as the guidance for the wider public of the National Institute for Health and Clinical Excellence in the UK), or it may instead lean towards propaganda to condition people to buy and use some product often by heightening worries about health.

There are, however, some rules of thumb that may be usefully applied to screen health information from Web searches or in the media:

- *Trust new findings only if replicated.* Frequently repeated claims such as, for instance, that a newly identified protein in tomatoes reduces the risk of colon cancer by half, should be treated with great caution, not because the result arises from a flawed study (it could) but, as stressed many times in this book, because a causal link can only be established through replicated, separate, and concordant investigations. Replicated investigations means several different studies, not the result of the same study echoed with various delays by several different media.
- *Trust only findings qualified by their uncertainty.* We all prefer a black-and-white image of reality, if nothing else because decisions to be taken are perforce yes or no. Yet most often there is some margin of uncertainty in the results and black-and-white

descriptions hide an essential part of the relevant information. Dogmatic statements should be treated with caution.

- *Trust findings only if placed in context.* Enabling people, in professional as in ordinary life, to transform information into empowering knowledge implies that information is not isolated nor randomly connected to other elements, but placed in context. For example, findings of studies on the possible cancer risks from mobile phone use should be discussed in the context of other health effects, including the risk of car accidents from use while driving. This can be done within the text itself or by links to external references. Such contextualization is essential in developing the reader's personal appropriation and interpretation of information; it does not substitute for it nor should it try to do so.
- *Trust findings only if not framed as advertisements.* Advertising is a signal necessary to draw attention to the substance, i.e. new or important findings. In commercial, sales-promoting reporting, however, the roles are completely reversed, the advertisement being the substance. Selling genetic profiles on the Web pretending, based on questionable or no evidence, to predict which diseases you will suffer in the future, has become a profitable enterprise. A safe rule would be to ignore it altogether: by ignoring such ventures, you lose nothing and when sound evidence about genetic factors predisposing to a disease becomes available, you will learn of them anyway from other, non-commercial sources.
- *Trust findings and recommendations only if concordant.* This is perhaps the most crucial guiding rule. With information, as with most other circumstances in life, there is no free meal; there are low-cost fast meals but they are of unknown quality. It is only by taking the time and effort of cross-checking the information from different sources, carefully looking at details, that one can be reasonably confident about the quality and validity of the information.

Health systems and public health

The health system is the common name for the complex of all activities directly dealing with health, although in most, if not all, countries this ensemble is more a complicated aggregate of many component systems than a unique organization. Public health coordination, itself one of the components operated chiefly by central, regional, and local health authorities, frames and interrelates the systems of hospitals (public, private for profit, private non-profit), general practices, clinical specialists, prevention units, and all other health-related activities.

Administrators at all levels of the health system, as well as political decision makers, constantly face the issue of comparing benefits and costs of interventions and services. Economic analyses may focus on exploring different ways of performing the same intervention, for instance the same number of renal dialyses, in order to identify the least costly procedure (*cost-minimization analysis*). Or they may compare the cost and the result, in terms of a common outcome like prolongation of life, of different interventions such as renal dialysis versus kidney transplant (*cost-effectiveness analysis*). Finally, they may compare costs and benefits of different interventions for the same or different conditions (hypertension treatment or influenza immunization?) in monetary terms or in some measure of 'value' as perceived by individuals (*cost utility*). Epidemiologists intervene in these analyses by providing evidence on health benefits and ill effects as evaluated by systematic reviews of biomedical and epidemiological studies. The same standard of rigorous scrutiny applied to this evidence also needs to be used for assessing the economic evidence. Short of this there is no guarantee that the health of all, including the most vulnerable, will stay ahead of other societal interests, industrial, financial, or ideological.

Chapter 10

Epidemiology between ethics and politics

The ethics of epidemiological studies

The conduct of epidemiological studies poses ethical problems, particularly concerning the confidentiality of identifiable personal data and the use of stored blood samples to carry out genetic and other tests. To what extent can data in documents which clearly identify the individual, such as birth and death certificates, medical and prescription records, or employment records, be consulted for epidemiological research purposes? It has been the practice until the relatively recent past that epidemiologists would freely access these data, under a simple clause of personal engagement to guarantee that the person would not be identified by other parties. This clause would permit, for instance, the use of prescription records to form a cohort of subjects who used a drug suspected to induce kidney cancer as a side effect and, second, establishing, by linking the subjects' names to a mortality register, whether this cohort experienced a particularly high rate of kidney cancer. This type of practice has since come under criticism. It is argued that in all circumstances the consent of the individual is required to make the documents available for research purposes, the exception being a public health emergency, such as an epidemic, that necessitates rapid consultation of identifiable personal records. It is not only the ethical principle of *doing good and not doing harm* that needs to be respected by protecting the confidentiality of personal data, but also the principle of *autonomy*. Autonomy, i.e. freedom of self-determination, dictates that the individual to whom the personal data belong has, not exclusively, but certainly before anyone else, the right to decide whether and how the data can be used.

Rigid adherence to these principles may have the simple consequence of making epidemiological research impossible. Dead people cannot give consent and living people may be nearly impossible to trace and ask for consent many years after the documents of interest were produced. Ethics experts, national regulators, and international institutions such as the World Health Organization have taken different stances in respect to these issues. In some countries, it proves difficult to link documents because the personal identifiers, for example names or social security numbers, are deleted or masked. Roundabout ways of achieving the link without knowledge of the identity of the person may exist, but they are cumbersome and, worse, they may entail frequent errors, making studies unreliable. In general, however, the trend is towards regarding an epidemiological investigation even without consent as permissible provided that (a) an ethics committee independent of the researchers proposing the study and including lay people has approved the research; and (b) explicit and strict conditions are respected in the consultation and linkage of the documents.

Even more ethically problematic are the issues raised by the recent establishment of repositories of biological specimens, for instance blood, on which a theoretically limitless number of old and new biochemical and genetic tests can be performed. The very purpose of these repositories is to permit tomorrow epidemiological investigations that may improve our understanding of diseases using tests not yet available today. For this reason, it is impossible to ask the person who donates the blood to consent to research that even the investigator cannot yet specify. General consent 'for medical research' is too wide to be regarded as 'informed' and it may also induce refusals. It may, however, be acceptable as consent to the storage of the blood in the repository provided it is accompanied by the clause that each actual use of the blood will occur within a research project approved by an ethics committee. It will then behove the ethics committee to judge, depending on the nature of the project, whether or not it is necessary to go back to the subjects and obtain their consent. This may not be demanded for a study of breast cancer risk, but it may be for a project investigating the hypothesis that some genes are associated with proneness to commit crime. Similar issues arise for blood or other biological specimens collected from patients in hospitals and stored when later uses are outside research on the disease or diseases of the patient.

Finally, very delicate problems arise when moving from observational to intervention studies. What should be the comparison treatment in a randomized trial testing a new preventive vaccine in a country with poor health services? The best current vaccine or a placebo, given the fact that in that country many or most people do not receive vaccines anyway? Although 'realistic', the latter option appears very debatable because it accepts different ethical standards depending on who is going to be included in a trial: if the same or a similar experiment were to be carried out in a developed country (maybe the very one producing the medication), the use of a placebo instead of the best existing medication would not be accepted. Local adaptations of study designs are admissible, but bending of basic moral principles of universal value are not acceptable for a third general ethical principle, *justice*. Basic ethical principles for medical and health research are outlined in the 'Declaration of Helsinki', a document periodically revised by the World Medical Association and first drafted in the aftermath of World War II to prevent the repetition of the criminal experiments practised on the camp inmates by the Nazis.

As a rule, all study protocols have to be approved by an ethics committee, typically composed of a dozen health professionals, ethics specialists, and lay people independent of the researchers proposing the study. Projects that involve only completely anonymous data may not be subject to ethics committee approval if the procedures satisfy the requirements of the data-protection authorities. A universally accepted principle is that a project which is scientifically invalid, hence incapable of producing reliable information, is automatically unethical and not acceptable. The requirement is crystal clear but its application is often imperfect. Study protocols may arrive on the desk of the ethics committee without previous evaluation of their scientific validity by an expert committee, and the ethics committee has to act in a dual role of assessing both the scientific aspects, a task for which it has at best limited competence, and the ethical aspects. This is still the situation prevailing in many countries. It affects epidemiology in particular, as even basic literacy in the subject is thin and ethics committees may not clearly grasp the distinctions, entailing sharp differences in ethical requirements, between observational studies with anonymous data, observational studies with personal identifiable data, and intervention studies such as randomized population trials.

Justice and health

Whatever the type of study, the ethics committee's task focuses on guaranteeing the protection of the subjects included in the investigation. The committees rarely discuss to what extent a study responds to the health needs of the country where it is conducted, an issue particularly relevant for developing countries that implies but goes beyond ethics into the politics of research and health. Political choices in these domains must first of all confront the dramatic inequalities existing between developed and developing countries. By far the largest proportion of biomedical research funds is spent on diseases affecting the minority of the world population (less than one-fifth) living in the developed world.

According to some estimates, 10% of the total world burden of diseases attracts 90% of the biomedical research funds (the so-called '90/10 divide'). Similarly, almost 90% of the money destined for health care is spent in developed countries and only 10% in the developing countries, where the great majority of humankind lives.

Although they are not the only determinants of health, these huge inequalities in investment and current expenditure involve vast disparities in health. A newborn in Africa can expect – if today's conditions do not improve – to live on average 30 years less than a newborn in North America or Europe. A child born in a country like Angola is more than 70 times more likely to die in the first few years of life than a child born in Norway, and a woman giving birth in sub-Saharan Africa is 100 times more likely to die in labour than a woman in a rich country. Early life and premature death is not only frequent in developing countries but may often be 'invisible', as noted in Chapter 9. In India, only one-third of deaths are accurately registered and for only one-third of them is the cause recorded.

That the sheer chance of being born in a developed rather than in a developing country makes such huge differences in life span and healthy life is a blatant social injustice, all the more in a world that has never been as wealthy as today.

Figure 17 shows the vast divergence between a sustained increase in the income per person in a number of the most developed countries of the world and the quasi stagnant amounts of per capita transfers for economic development and welfare assistance to the developing countries during the 40 years between 1960 and the end of the 20th century. The trend in the new century has, however, been more favourable, particularly for the specific sub-sector of health assistance, notably thanks to the inflow of private donations from major charities. Against this background, the United Nations fixed, in

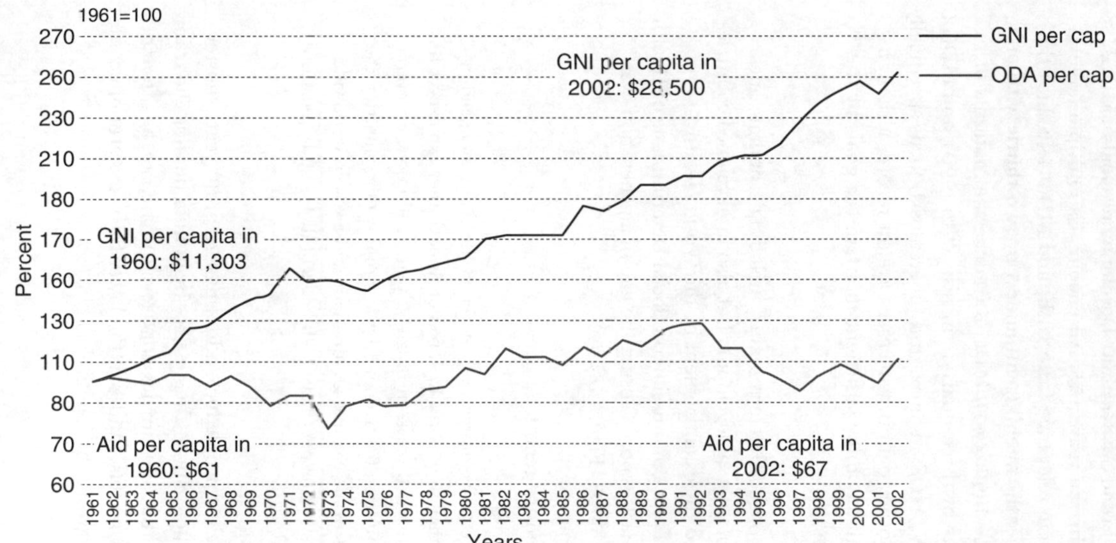

17. Between 1960 and 2002, the inflation-adjusted Gross National Income per capita (upper curve) of 22 high-income donor countries increased by 150%, while the amount donated to recipient countries as ODA (Official Development Assistance, lower curve) progressed by only 30% (in the most recent years, a partial correction of this widening gap has intervened)

2000, eight broad 'Millennium Development Goals' (MDGs) to be attained by the year 2015. All encompass multiple targets and have some relevance for health; and MDG 4 (reduce the number of deaths in children under 5 by two-thirds with respect to the 1990 level), MDG 5 (reduce the maternal mortality rate by three-quarters in respect to 1990), and MDG 6 (combat HIV/AIDS, malaria, and tuberculosis) focus specifically on health. So far, definite successes are on record, although at a pace unlikely to be sufficient to attain the goals by the 2015 deadline.

The key role of social determinants, including economic ones, for health not only in developing but also in developed countries has prompted the establishment by the World Health Organization of a Commission on Social Determinants of Health, whose landmark report 'Closing the gap in a generation' was published in 2008 (Figure 18).

To quote from the report:

> Our children have dramatically different life chances depending on where they were born. In Japan or Sweden they can expect to live more than 80 years; in Brazil 72 years; and in one of several African countries, fewer than 50 years. And within countries, the differences in life chances are dramatic and are seen worldwide. The poorest of the poor have high levels of illness and premature mortality.

In fact, homeless people have a life span 20 or 30 years shorter than their fellow citizens living close by in their homes. The report also stresses that in countries at all levels of income, health and illness follow a social gradient: the lower the socio-economic position, the worse the health.

Commission on Social Determinants of Health **FINAL REPORT**

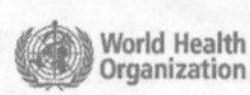

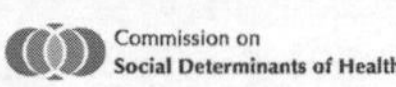

Closing the gap in a generation

Health equity through action on the social determinants of health

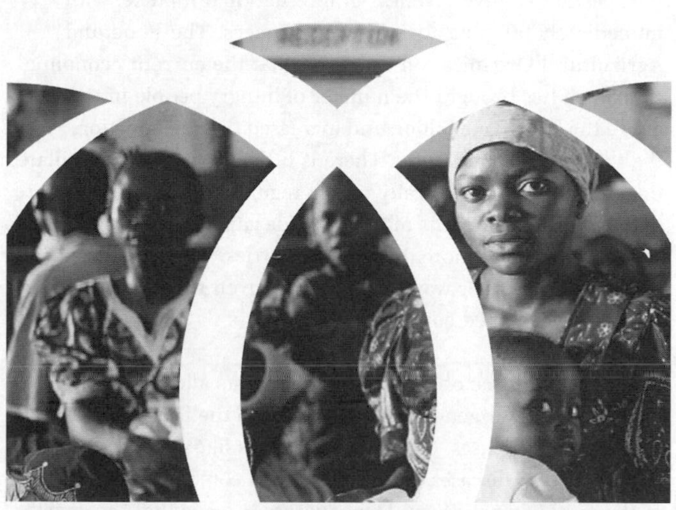

18. The 2008 Final Report of the World Health Organization Commission on Social Determinants of Health

Health without limits?

Within a society, disease has always mobilized at the same time the care of the sick and powers, natural, religious, magic, to fight disease. In the wake of the 17th century's scientific revolution, both care for the patients and powers intended to fight disease became slowly but steadily based on scientific and technical knowledge. Two centuries of development of industrial capitalism produced a further gradual transformation in disease care, treatment, and prevention, reaching in the second half of the 20th century the stage of a mature 'health industry', today one of the largest economic sectors in developed countries. Lately this has become, like most other sectors of the economy, tied to the speculative inventiveness of international finance, with immediately tangible adverse consequences. The Food and Agricultural Organization estimates that the current economic slowdown has brought the number of hungry people in the world above the bar of one billion and increased their proportion within the total world population. There is little doubt that unregulated finance, and more generally poorly regulated market forces, are important determinants of today's wide gaps in health conditions within and, much more, between countries. They are also responsible in other ways for a profit-driven rush to expanding health in developed countries.

One example is the offer via the Web of tests alleged to tell you whether your genes make you liable to the future occurrence of particular diseases. Common conditions like cancer, cardiovascular diseases, or diabetes are of course prime targets of the marketing strategy. The only sure thing is that the genetic tests are feasible and that you have to pay for them. How accurately they predict whether a disease will occur is for most of them neither declared nor known, and when the disease will occur is totally unknown. To advertise this approach as 'prevention' is mystifying because, in addition, for several conditions such as many cancers there is no well-established preventive measure even if one were to know with absolute certainty that the disease will occur. A second example is disease-mongering, the widening of the definition of treatable diseases so that even the mildest and most dubious cases receive medical treatment. Variants of normal behaviours are then classified as diseases requiring treatment, like the condition of restless leg or generic female sexual dysfunction.

Both these examples have common traits. Under the thin cover of complying with the 'right of people to know', they actually promote, for the sake of profit, dependency and suppression of critical judgement, of doctors by persuading them to prescribe drugs for people who could do without; of citizens by making them hungry for more tests, medical examinations, and medical remedies to pursue the mirage of unlimited health. These unhealthy trends go counter to the empowerment of people. A psychologist might say that they actually foster an 'infantile regression' among people by subtly fuelling fear and the need for continuous reassurance against it.

Epidemiology for justice in health

A card-carrying epidemiologist once said, 'today epidemiology is needed everywhere in medicine and public health'. Although formulated by an interested party, the statement is essentially correct. One major consequence is that no single person can competently master all or most areas of contemporary epidemiology and epidemiologists become specialized in particular fields of the discipline. Thus it is common to hear of genetic, environmental, social, cardiovascular, cancer, and paediatric epidemiology, and many other fields. Whatever their speciality, all epidemiologists share a common core of methods of investigation, of which this book has attempted to give a bird's-eye view, and a population perspective of health.

The term 'population', the trademark of epidemiology, however, covers two distinct aspects. First, population is the working tool of epidemiology, which uses populations to investigate diseases and health in the same way as other research uses mice, hamsters, or cell systems. The second aspect is people awaiting the reduction of their burden of diseases, and this may happen only to the extent that epidemiological research results are translated into effective interventions. Should epidemiologists use populations as expedient tools for science and do nothing about populations as targets for interventions simply because it is not their job as researchers? In academic circles this attitude is not uncommon: results of epidemiological research are best left at the door of colleagues in public health practice and of decision makers, allowing them to use the findings or not, as and when they see fit.

This attitude is objectionable on logical and ethical grounds. It contradicts the claim, very often advanced when requesting funds for epidemiological research, that because epidemiology directly studies humans, it can contribute more immediately than other biomedical research, for example experiments in the laboratory, to people's health.

It also deviates from the ethical principle that Immanuel Kant (Figure 19) formulated in neat terms at the time of the Enlightenment: any human should never be regarded only as a means, as would be the case if populations were considered by epidemiologists only as research instruments. Ensuring that results of research are effectively translated into benefits for all people, reducing the social injustices in health, demands an active involvement which may take variable forms, from assistance to full participation in decision making, to social critiques, and to advocacy initiatives. There is no room for confusion between this involvement and the duty of scientific impartiality: when one's ethical and political values are openly declared, scientific impartiality and judgements become well

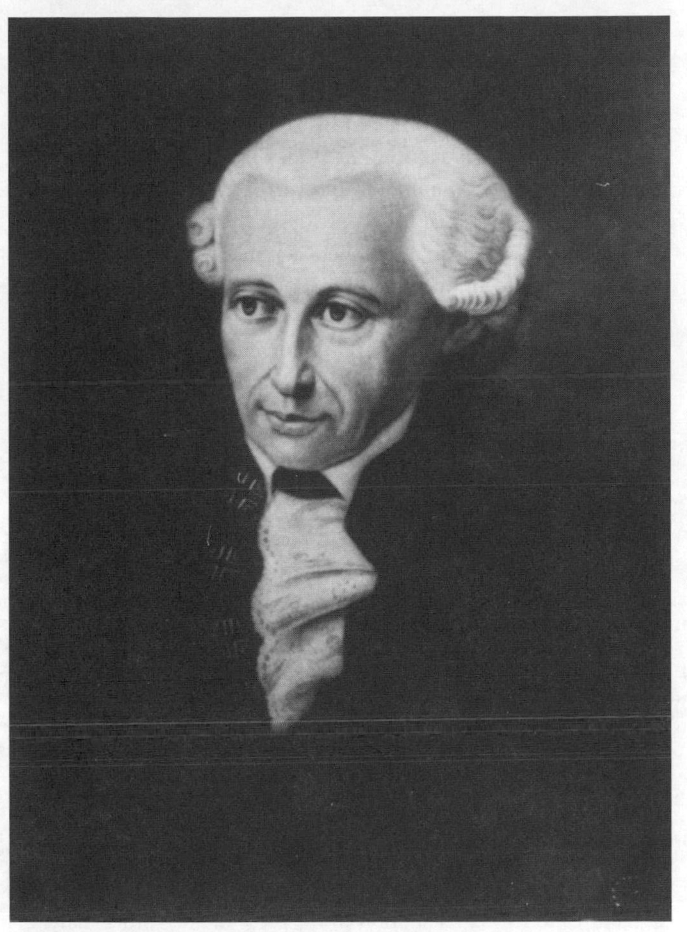

19. Immanuel Kant (1724–1804)

separated from the value judgements inherent in any advocacy or involvement in policy making.

Epidemiology has evolved as a response to diseases in society and is not only the product of technical and scientific developments but, as for any other science, reflects to a variable extent the ideas prevailing in society at different historical times. Today, personal liberty for everybody is a dominant idea, value, and aspiration in society. However, it cannot be 'for everybody' if it is not at least approximately an 'equal liberty', without the huge differences in power and resources that exist between individuals. Among the resources that feed individual freedom, health is the most basic; our direct experience teaches us that without health personal freedom is severely restricted. Thus advancing justice in health by minimizing health inequalities within and between countries is the common aim of all streams of epidemiology and the acid test of its value to health. As John Rawls put it: '*Justice* is the first virtue of social institutions, as *truth* is of systems of thought'. Both are guiding lights for epidemiologists.

References

Every chapter of the book reflects concepts and methods presented in the volumes listed in the Further reading section. Here key references are quoted specific to the narrative material and to the examples of each chapter, enabling the interested reader to locate their sources.

Chapter 1

M. G. Reynolds, B. H. Anh, V. H. Thu, J. M. Montgomery, D. G. Bausch, J. J. Shah et al., 'Factors associated with nosocomial SARS-CoV transmission among healthcare workers in Hanoi, Vietnam, 2003', *BMC Public Health* 6 (2006), 207–16.

R. Porter, *The Greatest Benefit to Mankind* (HarperCollins, 1997).

R. Saracci, 'Introducing the history of epidemiology', in J. Olsen, R. Saracci, and D. Trichopoulos (eds.), *Teaching Epidemiology*, 3rd edn. (Oxford University Press, 2009), pp. 1–19.

A. Morabia (ed.), *History of Epidemiologic Methods and Concepts* (Birkhäuser Verlag, 2004).

C. Buck, A. Llopis, E. Najera, and M. Terris (eds.), *The Challenges of Epidemiology: Issues and Selected Readings* (PAHO, 1988).

M. Porta (ed.), *A Dictionary of Epidemiology* (Oxford University Press, 2008), p. 81.

J. N. Morris, *Uses of Epidemiology*, 2nd edn. (Livingstone, 1964).

Chapter 2

World Health Organization, *Basic Documents*, 46th edn. (World Health Organization, 2007), p. 1.

A. S. Fauci, E. Braunwald, D. L. Kasper, S. L. Hauser, D. L. Longo, J. L. Jameson, and J. Loscalzo, *Harrison's Principles of Internal Medicine*, 17th edn. (McGraw-Hill, 2008).

World Health Organization, *International Classification of Diseases* (http://www.who.int/classifications/icd/en/, accessed 2009).

Chapter 3

J. Perlea, *Causality*, 2nd edn. (Cambridge University Press, 2009).

S. Greenland (ed.), *Evolution of Epidemiologic Ideas: Annotated Readings on Concepts and Methods* (Epidemiology Resources, 1987).

These two references are also directly relevant to Chapter 4.

Chapter 4

Royal College of Physicians, *Smoking and Health* (Pitman, 1962).

Advisory Committee to the Surgeon General of the Public Health Service, *Smoking and Health* (US Department of Health, Education and Welfare, 1964).

A. Bradford Hill, 'The environment and disease: Association or causation?', *Proc R Soc Med* 58 (1965), 295–300.

G. Rose, 'Sick individuals and sick populations', *Int J Epidemiol* 14 (1985), 32–8.

G. Rose, *Rose's Strategy of Preventive Medicine*, with a commentary by K. T. Khaw and M. Marmot (Oxford University Press, 2008).

R. Pearl, 'Tobacco smoking and longevity', *Science* 87 (1938), 216–17.

R. Doll and A. Bradford Hill, 'Smoking and carcinoma of the lung', *BMJ* ii (1950), 739–48.

E. L. Wynder and E. A. Graham, 'Tobacco smoking as a possible etiologic factor in bronchogenic carcinoma: A study of six hundred and eighty-four proved cases', *JAMA* 143 (1950), 329–36.

M. L. Levin, H. Goldstein, and P. R. Gerhardt, 'Cancer and tobacco smoking: A preliminary report', *JAMA* 143 (1950), 336–8.

R. Doll, R. Peto, K. Wheatley, R. Gray, and I. Sutherland, 'Mortality in relation to smoking: 40 years' observations on male British doctors', *BMJ* 309 (1994), 901–11.

R. Doll, R. Peto, J. Boreham, and I. Sutherland, 'Mortality in relation to smoking: 50 years' observations on male British doctors', *BMJ* 328 (2004), 1519–27.

International Agency for Research on Cancer, *Tobacco Smoke and Involuntary Smoking* (International Agency for Research on Cancer, 2004).

Chapter 5

T. Francis et al., 'An evaluation of the 1954 Poliomyelitis Vaccine Trials, Summary Report', *Am J Publ Health* 45 (1955), 1–63.

F. M. Sacks, G. A. Bray, V. J. Carey, S. R. Smith, D. H. Ryan, S. D. Anton et al., 'Comparison of weight-loss diet with different compositions of fat, protein and carbohydrates', *N Engl J Med* 360 (2009), 859–73.

Medical Research Council, 'Streptomycin treatment of pulmonary tuberculosis', *BMJ* ii (1948), 769–82.

The Gambia Hepatitis Study Group, 'The Gambia Hepatitis Intervention Study', *Cancer Res* 47 (1987), 5782–7.

G. D. Kirk, E. Bah, and R. Montesano, 'Molecular epidemiology of human liver cancer: Insights into etiology, pathogenesis and prevention from the Gambia, West Africa', *Carcinogenesis* 27 (2006), 2070–82.

R. Doll, R. Peto, J. Boreham, and I. Sutherland, 'Mortality in relation to smoking: 50 years' observations on male British doctors', *BMJ* 328 (2004), 1519–27.

The Alpha-Tocopherol, Beta-Carotene Cancer Prevention Study Group, 'The effect of vitamin E and beta carotene on the incidence of lung cancer and other cancers in male smokers', *N Engl J Med* 330 (1994), 1029–35.

M. J. Barry, 'Screening for prostate cancer: The controversy that refuses to die', *N Engl J Med* 360 (2009), 1351–4.

Chapter 6

E. Riboli, K. J. Hunt, N. Slimani, P. Ferrari, T. Norat, M. Fahey et al., 'European Prospective Investigation into Cancer and Nutrition (EPIC)', *Public Health Nutrition* 5 (6B, 2002), 1113–24.

C. A. Gonzalez, 'The European Prospective Investigation into Cancer and Nutrition (EPIC)', *Public Health Nutr* 9 (1A, 2006), 124–6.

J. Danesh, R. Saracci, G. Berglund, E. Feskens, K. Overvad, S. Panico et al., 'Epic-Heart: The cardiovascular component of a prospective study of nutritional, lifestyle and biological factors in 520,000 middle-aged participants from 10 European countries', *Eur J Epidemiol* 22 (2007), 129–41.

J. Olsen, M. Melbye, S. F. Olsen, T. I. A. Sørensen, P. Aaby, A. N. Nybo Andersen et al., 'The Danish National Birth Cohort: Its background, structure and aim', *Scand J Public Health* 29 (2001), 300–7.

UK Biobank, at http://www.ukbiobank.ac.uk, accessed 2009.

M. J. Pencina, R. B. D'Agostino Sr, M. G. Larson, J. M. Massaro, and R. S. Vasan, 'Predicting the 30-year risk of cardiovascular disease: The Framingham heart study', *Circulation* 119 (2009), 3078–84.

A. Morabia and R. Guthold, 'Wilhelm Weinberg 1913 large retrospective cohort study: A rediscovery', *Am J Epidemiol* 165 (2007), 727–33.

I. J. Selikoff, E. C. Hammond, and J. Churg, 'Asbestos, smoking and neoplasia', *JAMA* 204 (1968), 104–10.

Chapter 7

R. Macbeth, 'Malignant disease of the paranasal sinuses', *J Laringol* 79 (1965), 592–612.

A. L. Herbst, H. Ulfelder, and D. C. Poskanzer, 'Association of maternal stilbestrol therapy with tumor appearance in young women', *N Engl J Med* 284 (1971), 878–81.

J. T. Boyd and R. Doll, 'A study of the aetiology of carcinoma of the cervix uteri', *Brit J Cancer* 18 (1964), 419–34.

N. Munoz, F. X. Bosch, S. de Sanjosé, L. Tafur, I. Izarzugaza, M. Gili et al., 'The causal link between human papilloma virus and invasive cervical cancer: A population-based case-control study in Colombia and Spain', *Int J Cancer* 52 (1992), 743–9.

E. L. Franco, F. Coutlée, and A. Fernczy, 'Integrating human papillomavirus vaccination in cervical cancer control programmes', *Public Health Genomics* 12 (2009), 352–61.

The Wellcome Trust Case Control Consortium, 'Genome-wide association study of 14,000 cases of seven common diseases and 3,000 shared controls', *Nature* 447 (2007), 661–78.

Chapter 8

P. Vinten-Johansen, H. Brody, N. Paneth, S. Rachman, and M. Rip, *Cholera, Chloroform, and the Science of Medicine: A Life of John Snow* (Oxford University Press, 2003).

J. Müller-Nordhorn, S. Binting, S. Roll, and S. N. Willich, 'An update on regional variation in cardiovascular mortality within Europe', *Eur Heart J* 29 (2008), 1316–26.

A. Keys, *Seven Countries: A Multivariate Analysis of Death and Coronary Heart Disease* (Harvard University Press, 1980).

A. Bruneau and C. Duchesne, 'Outbreak of mumps, Montreal, October 1998 to March 1999, with a particular focus on a school', *Canada Communicable Disease Report* 26 (2000), 69–71.

C. Fraser, C. A. Donnelly, S. Cauchemez, W. P. Hanage, M. D. Van Kerkhove, T. D. Hollingsworth et al., 'Pandemic potential of a strain of Influenza A(H1N1): Early findings', *Science* 324 (2009), 1557–61.

M. Marmot and P. Elliott, 'Coronary heart disease epidemiology: From aetiology to public health', in M. Marmot and P. Elliott (eds.), *Coronary Heart Disease Epidemiology: From Aetiology to Public Health*, 2nd edn. (Oxford University Press, 2005), pp. 4–7.

A. Lopez, C. AbouZar, K. Shibuya, and L. Gollogly, 'Keeping count: Births, deaths, and causes of death', *Lancet* 370 (2007), 1744–6.

D. M. Parkin, S. L. Whelan, J. Ferlay, L. Teppo, and D. B. Thomas, *Cancer Incidence in Five Continents*, Vol. VIII (International Agency for Research on Cancer, 2003).

National Center for Health Statistics, *National Health and Nutrition Examination Survey* (http://www.cdc.gov/nahnes/, accessed 2009).

R. Saracci and P. Vineis, 'Disease proportions attributable to environment', *Environ Health* 6 (2007), 38–41.

World Health Organization, *Global Burden of Disease* (http://www.who.int/healthinfo/global_burden_disease/en/index.html, accessed 2009)

Chapter 9

P. Juni, L. Nartey, S. Reichenbach, R. Sterchi, P. A. Dieppe, and M. Egger, 'Risk of cardiovascular events and Rofecoxib: Cumulative meta-analysis', *Lancet* 364 (2004), 2021–9.

C. M. Rembold, 'Number needed to screen: Development of a statistic for disease screening', *BMJ* 317 (1998), 307–12.

P. Vineis, P. Schulte, and A. J. McMichael, 'Misconception about the use of genetic tests in populations', *Lancet* 357 (2001), 709–12.

G. Rose, *Rose's Strategy of Preventive Medicine*, with a commentary by K. T. Khaw and M. Marmot (Oxford University Press, 2008).

C. P. Cannon, 'Can the polypill save the world from heart disease?', *Lancet* 373 (2009), 1313–14.

P. Martens and A. J. McMichael, *Environmental Change, Climate and Health: Issues and Research Methods* (Cambridge University Press, 2002).

A. McMichael, S. Friel, A. Nyong, and C. Corvalan, 'Global environmental change and health: Impacts, inequalities, and the health sector', *BMJ 336* (2008), 191–4.

National Health Service, *National Institute for Health and Clinical Excellence (NICE)* (http://www.nice.org.uk/, accessed 2009).

M. F. Drummond, B. O'Brien, G. L. Stoddart, and G. W. Torrance, *Methods for the Economic Evaluation of Health Care Programmes* (Oxford University Press, 1997).

Chapter 10

T. Hope, *Medical Ethics: A Very Short Introduction* (Oxford University Press, 2004).

Council for International Organizations of Medical Sciences (CIOMS), *International Ethical Guidelines for Epidemiological Studies* (CIOMS, 2009).

United Nations, *Millennium Development Goals* (United Nations, 2000).

World Health Organization Commission on Social Determinants of Health, *Closing the Gap in a Generation* (World Health Organization, 2008).

Food and Agricultural Organization, *The State of Food Insecurity in the World* (Food and Agricultural Organization, 2009).

P. Vineis and R. Saracci, 'Gene–environment interactions and public health', in R. Detels, R. Beaglehole, M. A. Lansing, and M. Gulliford (eds.), *Oxford Textbook of Public Health* (Oxford University Press, 2009), vol. 3, pp. 957–70.

D. H. Moynihan, 'The fight against disease mongering: generating knowledge for action', *PLOS Medicine* 3 (2006), e191.

I. Kant, in A. Zweig (ed.), *Groundwork for the Metaphysics of Morals* (Oxford University Press, 2003).
R. Saracci, 'Epidemiology: A science for justice in health', *Int J Epidemiol* 36 (2007), 265–8.
J. Rawls, *A Theory of Justice* (Oxford University Press, 1972), p. 3.

Further reading

Knowing epidemiology

This book should have helped the reader to move from having heard (perhaps) of epidemiology to knowing epidemiology by the acquisition of some familiarity with its language and ways of reasoning and operating. The essentials of epidemiological jargon being clear, it will also be possible to get a grip on the meaning of the many terms that could not be included in the book and can be found by consulting when necessary the volume by M. Porta (ed.), *A Dictionary of Epidemiology*, 5th edn. (Oxford University Press, 2008).

A fascinating illustration of imaginative and rigorous 'diagnostic reasoning', at the core both of epidemiology (at population level) and of clinical medicine (at the individual level) springs from the stories that the late medical writer Berton Roueché presented over several decades in *The New Yorker*. A highly readable selection is collected in B. Roueché, *The Medical Detectives* (Penguin Books/Plume, 1991).

Using epidemiology

Using epidemiology requires us to go beyond surface familiarity with the subject. It implies not only the ability to read and appreciate an epidemiological paper or report, as someone who knows epidemiology can do, but also the skill for scrutinizing its methods and critically assessing its results and conclusions. Health professionals not directly practising epidemiology need to possess this skill to a degree sufficient for gauging the relevance of epidemiological findings to their daily work in clinical medicine or public health. Given favourable individual circumstances, this objective might be attained even by a self-teaching endeavour. There is no way, however, that such skill can be acquired through a simple accumulation of readings. Advancing through successive steps must be accompanied by a number of practical exercises in statistical and epidemiological methods. Suitable introductory books to the former are: D. Altman, D. Machin, T. Bryant, and S. Gardner, *Statistics with Confidence*, 2nd edn. (Wiley-Blackwell, 2000) and S. A. Glantz, *Primer of Biostatistics*, 5th edn. (McGraw-Hill, 2002). For epidemiological methods, one may refer to R. Bonita, R. Beaglehole, and T. Kjellström, *Basic Epidemiology*, 2nd edn. (World Health Organization, 2006) and to K. J. Rothman, *Epidemiology: An Introduction* (Oxford University Press, 2002). A useful addition to the questions and exercises in these two books is the substantial set of exercises, with answers, presented in S. E. Norell, *Workbook of Epidemiology* (Oxford University Press, 1995).

A computer-assisted learning package for basic epidemiological methods has been prepared and tested by C. du Florey and is available at no cost at the website: http://www.dundee.ac.uk/~cdvflore/. The International Epidemiological Association (IEA) website (http://www.IEAweb.org) cites without commentary a number of other didactic packages.

Short intensive courses in epidemiological methods, one to four weeks long, are available in several countries, and a selection of these is quoted in the R. Bonita et al. book mentioned above. The IEA organizes courses in developing countries and sponsors the residential summer school of the European Educational Programme in Epidemiology (http://www.eepe.org).

Doing epidemiology

Progressing from using epidemiology to doing it means becoming a professional regularly carrying out epidemiological work either in research or in service activities, or both. Substantial training is required, formal through special courses as well as informal through actual practice, to reach this level of competence. A vast array of books is available, among which a few key references may be quoted, some of recent date and some less recent that have withstood the test of time. For statistical methods, a classic is P. Armitage, G. Berry, and J. N. S. Matthews, *Statistical Methods in Medical Research*, 4th edn. (Blackwell Science, 2002). Specific to statistical methods in epidemiology are the book by D. Clayton and M. Hills, *Statistical Models in Epidemiology* (Oxford University Press, 1993) and the two volumes by N. E. Breslow and N. E. Day, *Statistical Methods for Cancer Research* (International Agency for Research on Cancer, 1980 and 1987). Current epidemiological methods are comprehensively treated in K. J. Rothman, S. Greenland, and T. L. Lasch, *Modern Epidemiology*, 3rd edn. (Wolters Kluwer, 2008). Epidemiology in relation to broad classes of health and disease determinants, environmental, nutritional, and genetic, are covered respectively in D. Baker and M. J. Nieuwenhuijsen, *Environmental Epidemiology* (Oxford University Press, 2008), W. Willett, *Nutritional Epidemiology*, 2nd edn. (Oxford University Press, 1996), and L. Palmer, G. Davey-Smith, and P. Burton (eds.), *An Introduction to Genetic Epidemiology* (The Policy Press, 2009). Epidemiology in the clinical medicine context is developed in R.B. Haynes, D.L. Sackett, G. Guyatt, and P. Tugwell, *Clinical epidemiology: how to do clinical practice research*, 3rd edn. (Lippincott Williams & Wilkins, 2006), and randomized clinical trials are addressed in S. J. Pocock, *Clinical Trials, A Practical Approach* (Wiley, 1983).

A wide spectrum of topics, including epidemiology, pertinent to health and diseases in populations is surveyed in the three volumes of R. Detels, R. Beaglehole, M. A. Lansing, and M. Gulliford, *Oxford Textbook of Public Health*, 5th edn. (Oxford University Press, 2009); although some of the more general chapters may be accessible to the lay reader, this is a text for professionals.

Index

INTELLIGENCE

A Very Short Introduction

Ian J. Deary

Ian J. Deary takes readers with no knowledge about the science of human intelligence to a stage where they can make informed judgements about some of the key questions about human mental activities. He discusses different types of intelligence, and what we know about how genes and the environment combine to cause these differences; he addresses their biological basis, and whether intelligence declines or increases as we grow older. He charts the discoveries that psychologists have made about how and why we vary in important aspects of our thinking powers.

> 'There has been no short, up to date and accurate book on the science of intelligence for many years now. This is that missing book. Deary's informal, story-telling style will engage readers, but it does not in any way compromise the scientific seriousness of the book . . . excellent.'
>
> **Linda Gottfredson, University of Delaware**

> 'Ian Deary is a world-class leader in research on intelligence and he has written a world-class introduction to the field . . . This is a marvellous introduction to an exciting area of research.'
>
> **Robert Plomin, University of London**

www.oup.co.uk/isbn/0-19-289321-1